BASIC
LIMBIC SYSTEM
ANATOMY OF
THE RAT

BASIC LIMBIC SYSTEM ANATOMY OF THE RAT

Leonard W. Hamilton

Rutgers University
New Brunswick, New Jersey

PLENUM PRESS · NEW YORK AND LONDON

Library of Congress Cataloging in Publication Data

Hamilton, Leonard W
 Basic limbic system anatomy of the rat.

 Bibliography: p.
 Includes index.
 1. Limbic system — Anatomy. 2. Rats — Anatomy. I. Title. [DNLM: 1. Limbic system —
Anatomy and histology. WL307 H218b]
QL938.L55H35   599'.3233   76-46401
ISBN 0-306-30925-4

©1976 Plenum Press, New York
A Division of Plenum Publishing Corporation
227 West 17th Street, New York, N.Y. 10011

Printed in the United States of America

To Claudia and Erika

. . . But, as the world, harmoniously confused:
Where order in variety we see,
And where, though all things differ,
all agree.

— Pope

Preface

If this were a traditional textbook of neuroanatomy, many pages would be devoted to a description of the ascending and descending pathways of the spinal cord and several chapters to the organization of the sensory and motor systems, and, perhaps, a detailed discussion of the neurological deficits that follow various types of damage to the nervous system would also be included. But in the first draft of this book, the spinal cord was mentioned only once (in a figure caption of Chapter 2) in order to illustrate the meaning of longitudinal and cross sections. Later, it was decided that even this cursory treatment of the spinal cord went beyond the scope of this text, and a carrot was substituted as the model. The organization of the sensory and motor systems and of the peripheral nervous system have received similar coverage. Thus, this is not a traditional text, and as a potential reader, you may be led to ask, ''What's in this book for me?''

This book is directed primarily toward those students of behavior who are either bored or frightened by the medically oriented texts that are replete with clinical signs, confusing terminology, and prolix descriptions of the human brain, an organ which is never actually seen in their laboratories. I should hasten to add, however, that this text may also serve some purpose for those who read and perhaps even enjoy the traditional texts. Briefly stated, this book is designed to take the reader step-by-step through the structures and interconnections of the limbic system (broadly defined to include the olfactory system, the hypothalamus, and parts of the cortex and midbrain).

The decision to prepare a textbook of anatomy devoted strictly to the limbic system was spawned by frustration and sustained by hope. The frustration arose from students who had just earned As in their anatomy course but could not tell a septal lesion from the lateral ventricle and did not know whether the fasciculus retroflexus was a type of camera or a part of the cerebellum. Worse still was the discovery that there were no books to which I could refer them that answer their questions. As an illustration, one of the most respected and widely used textbooks of anatomy (Ranson and Clark, 1959) devotes only 11 out of more than 600 pages to the anatomy of the limbic system. Most of the currently available descriptions of the limbic system are available only in technical articles which are at best tedious and at worst incomprehensible to the novice.

The hope that the need for a fundamental textbook could be met arose from a graduate seminar which I developed in an attempt to acquaint the students of our psychobiology program with the essential aspects of the limbic system anatomy. I discovered that with the proper sequence of models, stained sections, and line drawings, it was possible for students to become conversant with the anatomy of the limbic system and to actually begin to make serious use of known anatomical connections in the design of their research projects. The same strategy has been adopted in the format of this text.

In most cases, the system being described is first outlined in general terms with several accompanying photomicrographs to familiarize the reader with the topographical characteristics of the area. The more detailed descriptions of the fiber projections are presented in line drawings that maintain a superficial similarity to the actual structures but are schematically simplified to allow the student to easily redraw them for study purposes. It is strongly suggested that the student reorganize the material in ways other than those presented as an aid to thoroughly understanding the various interconnections. Furthermore, it is suggested that the text be used in conjunction with a photographic atlas such as that of König and Klippel (1967) and, if possible, in conjunction with stained sections of the rat brain.

The references to individual articles are frequently of little direct importance for a general summary of the anatomical connections but become critical for the reader who wants to study a particular system in detail. With this in mind, the number of references within the text have been kept to a minimum and a more complete annotated bibliography for each chapter appears in the appendix.

Lest the reader gain the mistaken impression that I am in basic disagreement with the format of traditional texts, I should point out that the rationale of the present text is quite similar; it represents an attempt to provide a structural framework that will foster a better understanding of function. The major difference is that this text provides a structural framework that is aimed more toward molar behavior rather than to reflexive behavior, sensory systems, etc. During the past three or four decades, experimental studies have demonstrated that the structures of the limbic system play important roles in the mediation of such complex behaviors as feeding and drinking, sexual behavior, emotional behavior, and learning and memory. Accordingly, it has become increasingly important for those who are interested in these behaviors to have a concise description of the anatomy of the limbic system. This text is intended to provide such a description. Owing to the fact that virtually all of the behavioral experimentation being carried out has utilized the rat as a subject, this text is restricted almost exclusively to the rat brain. Although it would be desirable to provide a detailed treatment of the known functional relationships, the volume of such a treatment would likely conceal the anatomy without, I fear, shedding too much light. The last chapter, however, is devoted to a brief summary of functions to at least introduce the reader to the relevant literature.

It is an unfortunate fact that anatomical terminology and interconnections are sometimes difficult to learn and always easy to forget. One of the major reasons for this is the terminology. There are frequently multiple names for the same structure as well as multiple opinions as to what constitutes a particular structure. Consequently, there have been attempts to standardize the nomenclature (e.g., International Anatomical Nomenclature Committee). Unfortunately, the resulting standardized terminology is tedious and not in common usage. I have often pointed out to students that the drawings in the König and Klippel (1967) atlas provide an excellent study guide because it is easier to learn to recognize the structures than it is to learn the abbreviations of the Latin terminology. This is quite appropriate for an atlas, but it is probably not the best way to be introduced to an anatomical system. For more than a decade, I have been engaged in research projects involving the septal region, and I have yet to hear a colleague refer to the nucleus septi lateralis. This structure is, quite simply, the lateral septum. In view of this chasm between the appropriate terminology and that which is in common usage, I have chosen to use the more readily understood anglicized terminology at the risk of occasionally oversimplifying. Once the major structures have been learned, the need for more detailed terminology and subtle distinctions of substructures will be more readily appreciated. By the time the student has reached this level of sophistication, it will be a relatively simple matter to supplement this basic knowledge via the more precise experimental literature.

Finally, I should point out that I am not now, have never been, and almost certainly never will be a neuroanatomist. I am a biopsychologist with an almost insatiable desire to determine relationships between the brain and behavior. In most cases, I use anatomical manipulations in an attempt to learn something about behavior. In other cases, I use behavioral approaches to learn something about anatomy. Because of my bias toward the behavioral aspects, I may sometimes oversimplify or even overlook some of the nuances of anatomical connections. Hopefully, these shortcomings will be outweighed by my being able to present an understandable, yet fairly complete account of the anatomical systems that are of especial interest to behavioral researchers.

LEONARD W. HAMILTON

Acknowledgments

This book did not arise from any specific suggestion, nor was it the fulfillment of some long-term ambition. It is rather a spontaneous development of two forces that exert more control over my life than I sometimes care to admit: One of these is the inexplicable lure of trying to understand the brain and behavior; the other is my unabashed eagerness to teach others what little is known about this topic. Accordingly, I am indebted to those who have contributed to these forces.

The initial kindling of my interests in the neurosciences is easy to pinpoint. It was Professor S. P. Grossman's undergraduate course in physiological psychology at the University of Iowa. I am grateful not only for this initial exposure, but also for his patient guidance of my graduate training at the University of Chicago. He afforded me the opportunity to learn that research is fun.

I am also grateful to the students who have worked in my laboratory at Rutgers University, sharing the labors of my joys. In particular, Sal Capobianco, Tom Schoenfeld, Robin Timmons, Fred vom Saal, and Liz Worsham have contributed their energies, their ideas, and their enthusiasm to the research that indirectly led to the writing of this text. I am especially grateful to Robin Timmons for the numerous ideas relating to style, format, and organization that have improved the quality of communication in this text.

Throughout the years, my research projects have been supported by the U.S. Public Health Service, the Rutgers Research Council, Biological Sciences Support Grants, and, most recently, the Weight Watchers Foundation, Inc.

An author is always indebted to a typist who can turn a rough copy into flawless black and white. This is especially true if the manuscript contains strange vocabulary and is constantly interrupted by figures and italicizing. My appreciation goes to Libby Brusca.

Finally, I am grateful to my wife, Claudia, for her understanding of my commitments to the laboratory, and to my daughter, Erika, for the laughter in her eyes. It would be dishonest to say that the preparation of this book resulted in lost evenings, weekends, and vacations. These were, in fact, lost, but, in the absence of this project, they would as likely have been lost to other manuscripts or other experiments.

L.W.H.

Contents

A Brief History of the Study of Neuroanatomy

1

THE EARLY ANATOMISTS

It has been said that there is an **anatomical instinct** in man, perhaps even in animals (Singer, 1957). A working knowledge of anatomy can be very useful to predatory animals, and, in fact, some of the earliest cave paintings depict crude drawings of animals with arrows pointing to the region of the heart. Not too surprisingly, the two organs that have received the most sustained interest have been the heart and the brain—the two organs that represent the most vulnerable targets for attack. It was, perhaps, because of this common denominator that teachers such as Aristotle tended to view these organs as a functional pair; Aristotle believed that the brain served as a sort of radiator for cooling the blood.

The formal, recorded study of anatomy dates back at least to the third century B.C. The first anatomist to dissect both human and animal bodies (at least in public) was Herophilus (300 B.C.–250 B.C.), who has been called the Father of Anatomy. On the basis of his dissections, he divided the nerves into motor and sensory divisions and distinguished the cerebellum and the cerebrum. The most influential early anatomist appeared some 450 years later, when Galen (129–199 A.D.) wrote two treatises on anatomy that were to be used as irrefutable (or, at least, irrefuted) sources for several centuries. These important publications were followed by a period of well over a thousand years during which time the science of anatomy was at a standstill, perhaps even on the decline. This unfortunate state of affairs that existed throughout the so-called Dark Ages was primarily the result of the Christian view that the soul was of prime importance, the body being unworthy of study.

The long silence in the study of anatomy was finally broken by Vesalius (1514–1564), who is almost universally considered to be the most important anatomist in the history of this field. Vesalius combined the early work of Galen with the new art, which

1

emphasized both accuracy and detail. Although he duplicated many errors and misconceptions that were put forth by Galen, his drawings were excellent and included a large number of new contributions. His treatment of the nervous system in general was somewhat crude, but his treatment of the brain was excellent: his drawings clearly showed the caudate nucleus, the thalamus, the stria terminalis, the fornix, the hippocampus, the corpora quadrigemina, and the superior and middle cerebral peduncles. This degree of detail is especially impressive when one considers that he only had a few human corpses to work on and that several of these were badly decomposed or hurriedly dissected for legal reasons. Even without the restrictions that existed against human dissection, these detailed descriptions would have been impressive: the brain is a very soft, highly vascularized tissue that rather quickly decomposes unless preservative techniques are employed at the time of death or shortly thereafter.

The work of Vesalius set the stage for the continuing development of the science of anatomy. As the attitudes toward human dissection began to mellow and the Galenic texts began to be supplanted by modern data, the descriptions of the **gross anatomy** of the brain were becoming quite detailed. But the early neuroanatomists realized that they were missing a great deal of information by not studying the structure of this complex organ in greater detail. Robert Hooke described cellular structure as early as 1665, using a crude microscope. The microscope was improved by Leeuwenhoek during the early part of the next century, and by 1850, the importance of cells was realized and the so-called **cell theory** came into general acceptance. Although the microscope was responsible for major advances in determining the detailed anatomy of a number of organ systems, brain tissue seemed particularly recalcitrant to being studied—thin sections of brain tissue appeared to be nothing more than homogeneous, translucent, gray blobs which yielded virtually no information about the substructure of the brain.

One of the most important milestones in the study of neuroanatomy was the development of histological procedures that made it possible to study this tissue microscopically. All sorts of staining procedures were attempted, and with the aid of rather crude microscopes, one of the fundamental characteristics of the nervous system became apparent: namely, that it is composed of rather long strands of protoplasm. This observation gave rise to a sometimes bitter controversy as to whether these strands represented portions of a continuous protoplasmic mass or were discrete cellular units which were intermeshed with each other. The major opponents in this controversy were Santiago Ramón y Cajal and Camillo Golgi, Golgi taking the view that the nervous system was a protoplasmic **syncytium.** This apparently simple question of structure could not be answered until a better staining procedure was developed. Ironically, Golgi developed a much improved staining procedure in the 1870s that allowed Cajal to demonstrate that the nervous system was, in fact, composed of discrete units, or neurons. In 1906, these two gentlemen shared the Noble Prize for their contributions leading to the adoption of the so-called **neuron doctrine.** Thus, it was less than 100 years ago that even this basic information about the units of the central nervous system became available. Viewed in this perspective, our present knowledge of the nervous system is a tribute to both the imagination and the hard labors of the twentieth century neuroanatomists.

Attempts to systematize the gross anatomical characteristics of the brain were being made at the same time that advances were being made at the microscopic level. In 1878, a

French physician named Pierre Paul Broca described the set of anatomically related structures that occupies the medial aspects of the cortical mantle. These structures—the subcallosal area, the gyrus fornicatus (including the gyrus cinguli and the uncus), and the parahippocampal gyrus—form a ring (**limbus**) around the inner border of the cortical mantle, an observation which led Broca to collectively term these structures **le grande lobe limbique** (see Fig. 1–1).

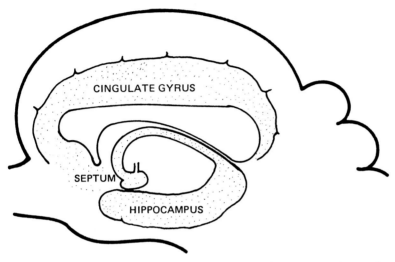

Fig. 1-1. The ring-like shape of the set of structures shown in the figure led Broca to use the term, *le grand lobe limbique*.

It should be pointed out that Kölliker had described these same structures in 1870, calling them the **rhinencephalon.** The term ''rhinencephalon'' means smell-brain and refers to the observation that these structures are in rather close juxtaposition to olfactory structures. Thus, there were two terms that came into common usage, one indicating structure, the other indicating presumed function.

TWENTIETH CENTURY ADVANCES

At the turn of the century, two American neuroanatomists made what may have been the most important technical advance in the study of the brain since the invention of the microscope. Horsely and Clark (1908) developed an accurate procedure for localizing brain structures in the intact organism. This procedure entails the use of a **stereotaxic instrument** that places the brain of the organism within a set of three-dimensional coordinates. The apparatus immobilizes the organism's head, usually by the insertion of specially adapted steel bars into the bony canals of the ear along with a jaw clamp that is usually designed to fit in back of the upper incisors (see Fig. 1–2). To the extent that the skull size and the location of the brain within the skull are nearly constant among the adult members of a particular species, it should be possible to localize any structure within this set of coordinates. This localization procedure utilizes the following three planes of reference:

1. A **horizontal** plane (H) is used to determine the height of a particular structure. Typically, the zero point is the interaural line (i.e., a line passing directly between the ears); all distances above that plane are given positive signs, while those below are given negative signs. The angle of this plane can vary depending on the height of the incisor bar.

2. A **lateral** plane (L) is used to determine the distance of structures from the midline (or **midsagittal** plane) of the brain. One set of planes, of course, includes the left half of the brain, while the other set includes the right half.

3. An **anterior–posterior** plane (AP), also called the **coronal** plane, is used to determine the distance of structures anterior or posterior to the interaural line, which is typically used as the zero point for this set of planes. Points anterior to this line are given positive signs while those posterior to the line are given negative signs. Both the lateral and the anterior–posterior planes are perpendicular to the horizontal plane.

This set of coordinates can be used to accurately locate any point, e.g., H = +1.5 mm; L = 0.8 mm; AP = −2.0 mm defines a point which is located 1.5 mm above, 0.8 mm lateral, and 2.0 mm behind the midpoint between the two ears. By experimentally locating stained brain sections within this system of coordinates, one can develop a **stereotaxic atlas** which can be used to facilitate the surgical destruction or the stimulation of a discrete area of the brain.

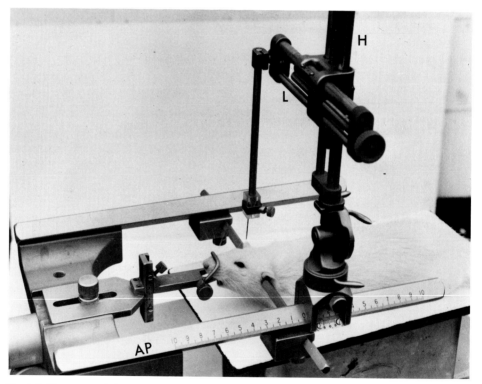

Fig. 1-2. The stereotaxic instrument was first developed by Horsely and Clark in 1908. The modern version shown here (David Kopf Instruments, Co.) is based on the same principles of using solid bony structures (e.g., the ear canals and the roof of the mouth) to precisely position the brain of the anesthetized rat within a set of three-dimensional coordinates. The horizontal (H), lateral (L), and anterior–posterior (AP) scales of the instrument are indicated.

For a period of about three decades following the invention of the stereotaxic instrument, neuroanatomists used this procedure to aid them in the investigation of the anatomy of larger animals (e.g., dog, cat, and monkey), while psychologists were using the smaller and less variable (due to selective breeding) rat for the investigation of behavioral variables. It was not until 1939 that these procedures were combined; Clark (1939) modified the Horsely-Clark instrument for use on the rat. Almost immediately, Hetherington and Ranson (1940) used the stereotactic procedure to produce highly localized damage within the hypothalamus and to demonstrate that the hyperphagia and obesity that followed damage to the base of the brain was attributable to the destruction of a small portion of the hypothalamus—the ventromedial nucleus. The combination of the adaptation of the stereotaxic instrument for use on the rat and the almost immediate publication of a paper showing the power of this technique for behavioral–anatomical studies paved the way for the subsequent rapid growth of our knowledge of the relationships between behavior and anatomy.

THEORETICAL APPROACHES

In order to define the orientation of this text, we must trace another line of historical developments in the area of behavioral–anatomical research that utilized the **ablation** procedure. The rationale of the ablation procedure is to damage a specific area of the nervous system and then to determine the functions which are lost. One of the more heroic efforts along these lines was the classic series of studies undertaken by Karl Lashley (e.g., 1950), who spent more than three decades attempting to determine the locus of memory. These experiments involved the somewhat crude technique of removing large areas of the cortex before testing the animal's memory of a particular task. The results of these experiments rather convincingly demonstrated that no area of the cortex is **essential** for learning or memory. This finding had the dual effect of diminishing the presumed importance of the cortex while suggesting (by default) that subcortical structures may be more important than previously believed.

At about the same time that Lashley was conducting his series of experiments, other developments were taking place that would further increase the interest in subcortical structures. It was gradually becoming apparent from anatomical studies that the relationship of these structures with the olfactory bulbs was less pronounced than originally believed (e.g., Herrick, 1933; Pribram & Kruger, 1954). Furthermore, clinical observations revealed that their involvement in emotional behaviors was much more pronounced than originally believed, findings leading Papez to speculate ''. . . that the hypothalamus, the anterior thalamic nuclei, the gyrus cinguli, the hippocampus, and their interconnections constitute a harmonious mechanism which may elaborate the functions of central emotion . . .'' (1937, p. 744). At about the same time that Papez published his largely speculative paper on the importance of subcortical structures in emotional behavior, Klüver and Bucy (1938) described a series of experiments in which extensive temporal lobotomies inflicted damage upon several of these subcortical structures in monkeys. The dramatic changes in behavior that followed this damage included a pronounced flattening of emotionality, with both fearful and aggressive responses being either absent or greatly diminished. These experimental and theoretical papers led to a surge of interest in the relationship of the subcortical structures to emotional behavior, and the term ''rhinencephalon'' was gradually replaced by the more descriptive term **limbic lobe.**

There occurred, then, in the late 1930s a convergence of ideas relating to the study of the relationship between the brain and behavior. The combination of technical advances in anatomy, the application of these techniques to behavioral studies, and the realization that so-called higher forms of behavior may be under the control of subcortical rather than cortical structures essentially set the stage for a new field of physiological psychology developed to investigate in detail the neural mechanisms that control behavior.

THE SCOPE OF THIS VOLUME

The present treatment of anatomy differs from the classic treatments of this subject matter in that it is directed primarily toward the student of psychobiology rather than toward the medical student. Accordingly, the well-defined anatomy of the spinal cord and cerebellum as it relates to the sensory and motor systems will not be presented. Nor will the relationships between the brain stem and vital functions (e.g., respiration, heart rate, etc.) be presented. The anatomy of the direct sensory projection areas and motor areas of the cortex and thalamus will be only broadly summarized as required. All of these circuits have been eloquently detailed in other sources, especially in the case of human anatomy (cf. Crosby, Humphrey, & Lauer, 1962; Ranson & Clark, 1959; Truex, 1969).

The present treatment will present the anatomical relationships of those areas which are most frequently of concern to the physiological psychologist; namely, those areas which appear to be involved in the control of regulatory behavior, reproductive behavior, emotional behavior, learning, and memory. In particular, the interrelationships between the classically defined limbic system structures, the olfactory system, the hypothalamus, parts of the thalamus, and parts of the midbrain will be described.

The anatomical descriptions will be based upon the brain of the rat for the simple reason that the rat is the subject of choice for most experiments conducted by physiological psychologists. Unfortunately, it has not been the traditional subject of choice for neuroanatomists (because of the small brain size), but in recent years its popularity in research has increased to such an extent that reasonably detailed accounts of the regions covered in this text are available in the experimental literature.

The photomicrographs used in this text were produced by using cresylviolet-stained brain sections as photographic **negatives.** As a result of this procedure, the unstained fibers appear dark in the final print.

Neuroanatomical Procedures and Terminology

2

INTRODUCTION

The study of neuroanatomy is at once a descriptive system of classification and a dynamic field of scientific inquiry. There are probably many reasons for applying names and descriptions to the (initially) subtle variations of the texture of the brain, not the least of which is man's apparently ancient penchant for naming and classifying the objects in his environment. But there are relatively few aspects of man's environment that have been named and classified to such an extent as has the brain. It is, therefore, fair to question the reasons for this degree of attention.

When viewed in an historical perspective (cf. Chapter 1), the major impetus for engaging in this tedious task of describing brain structures lies in the realization that this organ controls what is usually very complicated behavior. With this realization, the study of the brain is little different from the study of any other complex and wonderful machine. The observer is compelled to ask: What does it do? and How is it put together?

The answer to the first question will require an understanding of the dynamics of nature's boldest experiment—placing free-ranging organisms in a constantly changing and potentially dangerous environment. The answer to the second question will require an understanding of the intricacies of several billion individual units, each interconnected with as many as several thousand other units in a complicated fashion. Quite obviously, these questions will not be answered in detail, but the pursuit of the more general answers has provided the realm of scientific inquiry with its most intriguing subjects.

Almost every neuroscientist has at one time or another entertained the hope that the brain could be parcelled into discrete units, each of which would control a specific function. The incidence of this misconception reached almost epidemic proportion during the years that followed the modification of the stereotaxic instrument for use in the rat (Clark, 1939). This new technique appeared to offer an answer to the problem of lack of

7

specificity that had plagued earlier research using the extirpation procedure. But the small localized electrolytic lesions that could be produced by this technique did not solve the problem. Nor did the application of pharmacological compounds to the central nervous system or the use of sophisticated stimulation and recording techniques. Researchers are still faced with two perennial problems: There appear to be no discrete behaviors that are completely controlled by a single region of the brain, and there appear to be no discrete regions of the brain that are involved with only one category of behavior. Although this pair of problems has the advantage of guaranteeing the existence of research problems in the neurosciences, it frustrates the efforts to describe the interaction between behavior and the organ that is known to control that behavior.

Given these two problems, there are two systematic ways to determine the relationship between behavior and the brain. One is to produce a specific type of brain damage and assess the effects of this damage on all possible types of behavior, physiological functions, and perceptual abilities. Upon completion of this task, a new brain site could be selected and the process could be repeated. A second approach would be to select a specific behavior and assess the effects on it of damage inflicted upon all possible regions of the brain. Upon completion of this task, a new behavior could be selected and the process could be repeated. Either of these approaches would try the patience of the most dedicated researcher, and both are highly inefficient. Consequently, the approach has been to compromise, so that any particular investigator is likely to be interested in several different behaviors and/or several different regions of the brain.

Although it would be ideal to present an integrated treatise on structure and function, the many gaps in both the anatomical and behavioral data do not allow such an approach. This text is, therefore, aimed primarily toward providing a summary of anatomical connections with only brief references to function. Integral to understanding and appreciating the anatomical connections is a knowledge of both the neuroanatomical procedures and the terminology employed by researchers in this field.

NEUROANATOMICAL PROCEDURES

The modern study of neuroanatomy is an incredibly complex and multifaceted science that relies heavily upon a combination of theory, technology, art, and occasionally a bit of magic. A detailed discussion of the procedures and apparatus and interpretation of their use would go far beyond both the scope of this text and the expertise of the author. It may, however, be useful to review in very general terms the range and rationale of the procedures that are available. As will become apparent subsequently, there are a variety of procedures that are especially suited to particular research problems that may arise. Instructions for standard procedures may be found in a variety of sources, including Drury and Wallington (1967) and Wolf (1971). For an indication of the current state of the art, the reader is referred to an excellent series of articles in Nauta and Ebbesson's (1970) *Contemporary Research Methods in Neuroanatomy* (see Appendix, pp. 130–131).

In the first chapter it was noted that the brain is a very soft and somewhat nondescript tissue in its natural state. Although it is possible to identify major landmarks in an untreated brain, the application of procedures to harden and preserve the brain greatly facilitates gross observations and is absolutely essential for more detailed methods of histological analysis.

The substance of the brain is interwoven with a dense network of blood vessels and capillaries that help provide the somewhat unique metabolic requirements of that organ. The presence of coagulated blood and blood cells would severely hamper the observation of the detailed structure of the brain, so it is essential to remove the blood from the brain (desanguinate) prior to observation. In the case of small organisms such as the rat, this can be accomplished quickly and easily through direct intracardial perfusion. To perform this procedure, the rat is anesthetized and the chest cavity is opened to expose the heart. A hypodermic needle is inserted into the tip of the left ventricle of the heart and the right atrium in ruptured with a pair of sharp scissors. This opens the circulatory system so that the injection of isotonic saline under pressure (either gravity flow or via a syringe) flushes out the blood vessels and fills the entire system with saline. The purpose of using saline, of course, is to minimize the distortion and cellular damage that would result from drastic changes in osmotic pressure.

The simple replacement of the blood with saline accomplishes the purpose of clearing the tissue, but the cells of the brain would still undergo deterioration unless additional steps were taken to preserve the tissue. Toward this end, a solution of formalin and saline (formol saline) is injected through the left ventricle of the heart, replacing the saline that occupies the circulatory system. Within a few minutes, this preservative solution begins to harden the brain, which can then be carefully removed from the skull with a minimum of damage. (It should be pointed out that for detailed histological work, further precautions, such as chilling the perfusion solutions and using a buffered formalin solution, are necessary to further minimize distortion and destruction of cells.)

Upon removal of the brain from the skull, the brain can be stored in either a formol-saline solution or a 30% sucrose-formalin solution for periods ranging up to several years with little or no further deterioration. The sucrose-formalin solution in especially advised if the brain tissue is to be frozen for histological sectioning. The sucrose reduces the formation of large ice crystals, thereby minimizing damage to the thin sections of tissue (cf. Nauta & Ebbesson, 1970, Chapter 7).

GROSS OBSERVATION

The simplest method of studying the brain, gross observation and dissection, is also the best way to gain an appreciation of the major landmarks and relationships of various brain structures. An experienced eye can easily identify 50 to 100 structures, even in a brain as small as the rat brain. The relatively soft composition of the brain and the physical separation of various structures by sulci, by membranes, and by the ventricular system make the brain fairly easy to dissect. In one respect, the brain is a particular joy to the novice dissectionist—the old canon ''Always tease, never cut'' can be flagrantly violated. Although it is sometimes advisable to carefully tease away some of the surface structures to expose subcortical nuclei and fiber systems it is also quite instructive to slice through the brain to reveal the structures in cross section. Ideally, one should have at least four brains available for dissection. One of these should be dissected by removal of some of the surface structures, while the others should be carefully sliced (using a scalpel or razor blade) into thin (2–4 mm) sections taken in coronal, parasagittal, and horizontal planes, respectively. These tissue preparations can be preserved almost indefinitely in the formol-saline solution for future reference.

MICROSCOPIC OBSERVATION

Most of the available knowledge of the interconnections of brain structures has been gained through the aid of microscopic observations. Although it is possible to recognize fiber bundles and nuclear groups through gross observation, there are obvious limitations to this technique. As indicated in Chapter 1, the major difficulty encountered with early microscopic evaluation was the translucent nature of the brain tissue. Because of this, the search for better staining procedures has a long and sometimes colorful history.

CELL BODY STAINS

The Golgi Stain

One of the earliest and most useful staining procedures was that developed by Golgi in the 1880s. This procedure, which stains the entire cell body and its processes a golden brown color, has been especially useful in determining the complex structures of some of the cells of the central nervous system (e.g., cortical and cerebellar cells). For reasons that are still unknown, this staining procedure affects only a small, seemingly random proportion of the total cell population. If this were not the case, this currently valuable procedure would likely have been overlooked because of the crude technology that was available to Golgi. If all the cells of Golgi's thick tissue sections had been stained, the tissue would have been virtually opaque and microscopic analysis would have been impossible. (It should be noted that thick sections [100–300 μ] are required by this technique, the stain being incorporated into relatively thick blocks of tissue before slicing is undertaken.)

The Golgi technique represents one of the most important contributions to the histological study of the nervous system. In Chapter 1, the auspicious beginnings of this procedure were noted in that it led to the discovery that the central nervous system is composed of discrete cellular units. Remarkably, the exact procedures used by Golgi, as well as a number of variations, are still commonly used today for investigations ranging from synaptic ultrastructure to developmental neurology. Excellent accounts of the procedures and results of this technique may be found in Chapters 1, 2, 3, and 10 of Nauta and Ebbesson (1970).

Most of the techniques that have been developed since Golgi's time have capitalized on the fact that not all parts of the neuron show an equal affinity to certain types of chemicals. As an example, the fiber paths tend to attract certain classes of compounds while the cell bodies tend to attract other classes of compounds. This selective affinity for staining compounds has made it possible to stain thin sections of tissue so that the fiber tracts and nuclear groups are sharply contrasted on the basis of color or optical density or both.

The Cresylviolet Stain

One of the most common procedures for routine histological examination involves the use of an acidic solution of cresylviolet, which selectively stains the basic Nissl substance of the cell bodies, facilitating easy identification of nuclear groups. Because of the widespread use of this procedure and the fact that this method was used for the preparation of the material presented in the photomicrographs of this book, the procedures and rationale will be outlined in some detail. Rather than attempting to outline an exhaustive list of variations in technique, the procedures outlined here will be those that are routinely used in the author's laboratory. Most of the variations are a matter of preference and do not significantly alter the final result.

A simple and convenient procedure for preparing thin sections for staining is to use a freezing microtome. The brain is removed from storage in the sucrose-formalin solution and is carefully transected in the same plane in which the slices are to be made, i.e., a longitudinal section would be removed from one side for parasagittal sections and a cross cut (usually just in front of the cerebellum) would be made for coronal sections. This cut should be performed carefully because it provides the base for mounting on the stage of the microtome and will accordingly determine the precise orientation in which the cut will be made.

The block of tissue is then placed on the stage of the microtome and frozen into position with liquid carbon dioxide. For this particular stain, the sections are usually 30–50 μ thick, which is exquisitely thin relative to the procedures that were available to Golgi but crudely thick relative to the ultrathin sections that must be made for electron microscopy. The frozen sections are transferred to a 50% alcohol solution in an ice-cube tray or similarly compartmentalized container to keep the sections in the appropriate sequence.

Upon completion of slicing through all regions of interest, the sections are transferred to a gelatin solution and mounted on glass slides. The gelatin-soaked sections will stick to the slide, and further air-drying of the sections causes them to adhere firmly; this allows the tissue to be passed through the various staining solutions without danger of loss of the sections from the slides.

The air-dried sections are, of course, in a desiccated state and should be **rehydrated** somewhat gradually. Thus, the initial steps of the staining procedure involve passing the sections sequentially through 95% alcohol, 70% alcohol, and then water before entering the aqueous solution of cresylviolet. The **staining** solution impregnates the entire section, resulting in a uniformly dense, deep violet section of brain tissue in which no structures would be recognizable. The next step is to **differentiate** the sections by selectively removing the stain from the fiber tracts of the tissue. Before doing this, the sections must once again be dehydrated by being passed sequentially through 95%, 100%, and 100% alcohol. The dehydrated sections are placed in a bath of chloroform, which tends to dissolve the lipid of the myelinated fibers, removing the stain from the fiber surfaces in the process. As a result of this treatment, the fibers are once again translucent white in appearance and stand out in sharp contrast to the nuclear subdivisions that maintain the violet color in the Nissl substance of the cell bodies. The stained tissue is then passed through absolute alcohol for rinsing and clearing and is finally soaked in xylene to be permanently **fixed** in a stable condition. When the slides are removed from the xylene bath, a special tissue-mounting medium is dropped onto the sections and a glass cover slip is positioned over the sections. This protects the tissue from physical damage and seals it from the harmful effects of air. If all these steps are properly executed, the stained tissue is quite stable and can be saved for future study almost indefinitely.

In summary, the entire histological procedure entails the following steps: (1) desanguinating, (2) preserving and hardening, (3) freezing and sectioning, (4) mounting, (5) staining, (6) differentiating, (7) fixing, and (8) sealing. Most of these steps are common to the stains that are routinely used; therefore, they will not be outlined again in the following discussion of other staining procedures.

FIBER STAINS

Luxol Blue

The luxol blue stain is not frequently used as an exclusive fiber stain but is cited here because of its popularity as a **counterstain** along with cresylviolet (Kluver & Barrera, 1953). This procedure involves two staining processes in sequence. First, the tissue is stained with luxol blue (which stains myelin), and then with the cresylviolet cell stain (which stains the Nissl substance). The resulting sections show violet-colored nuclear groups with blue fibers interconnecting them. This not only aids in the microscopic examination of the material, but also yields sections that are superb from an aesthetic point of view.

Iron-Hematoxylin

One of the more widely used fiber stains is the iron-hematoxylin stain, which produces dense black fibers against a brown background. This stain was first developed by Weigert in the late 1800s (see Drury & Wallington, 1967). It involves staining in the hematoxylin solution followed by decoloration in a solution of potassium ferricyanide, which differentially removes the stain from the cell bodies while leaving the fibers darkly stained. Thus, the stain can be utilized as a counterpart to the cresylviolet stain, alternate sections being stained by each procedure. In some respects, it is easier to observe the details of both the nuclei and the fiber groups if one set of sections is stained with a cell stain and the other with a fiber stain, because the unstained components are optically less dense than if stained with a counterstain as in the Klüver-Barrera technique.

Silver Stains

Silver stains were developed as early as 1904 by Bielschowski and have been effectively used for many years to stain fiber systems. The basic procedure is remarkably similar to the photographic process although the underlying chemistry may be different. The first step is to impregnate the tissue with silver nitrate, forming the equivalent of a photographic emulsion. Then, the tissue is exposed to a reducing solution that forms an optically dense complex with the silver nitrate (the exact structure is unknown), leaving the fibers stained a dark brown to black color and the nuclear groups a lighter golden brown. The sections are then treated with sodium thiosulfate (fixer) and permanently mounted for future use.

SPECIALIZED FIBER STAINS

The staining procedures just described are representative of a wide variety of stains that have been developed. The search for new stains has been vigorously pursued not only to satisfy the scientific curiosity and aesthetic inclinations of the investigators, but more importantly to provide methods for a more detailed analysis of the structures of the central nervous system. Some of the stains (e.g., the Golgi stain) have been extremely useful because they provide a detailed view of the structure of individual cells. Stains like the cresylviolet stain are useful in outlining the morphological subdivisions of brain structures on the basis of cell size, cell density, organizational characteristics, etc. Fiber stains have been particularly useful in determining the connections between various nuclear subdivisions.

The limitations of some of these procedures became increasingly apparent as investigators attempted a fine-grained analysis of the systems. It is difficult, sometimes impossible, to trace long fibers from one region of the brain to another somewhat distant region and still be certain that the same fibers are being traced; there is always the possibility that fibers from other sources have joined those that are being traced, and it is difficult to ascertain whether fibers (especially small-diameter ones) are passing to or through a given nucleus.

A further limitation of these staining procedures is based on the pharmacological characteristics of the nerve fibers. The standard fiber stains or cell stains are nonspecific with respect to the chemistry of the neurons and therefore provide only a quantitative description of the central nervous system connections rather than a qualitative one. The remainder of this chapter will be devoted to a brief description of the specialized stains that have been developed to circumvent some of these limitations.

STAINS FOR DEGENERATING FIBERS

The most valuable addition to the arsenal of stains has been the modification of the silver stain to selectively stain fibers that are undergoing degeneration. Before considering these staining procedures, a brief discussion of degenerative processes per se may be useful.

Destruction of a neuron or transection of its long fiber processes can result in three basic types of degeneration.

One type of degeneration, termed **Wallerian** or **primary degeneration,** always occurs: the segment of the fiber that is disconnected from the supportive functions provided by the soma undergoes degeneration and is removed by the body's phagocytic processes. The time required for the completion of this process is a function of a number of variables, the most important of which is fiber size (large fibers degenerate more rapidly). In general, fibers of moderate size begin to show signs of degeneration within a few hours. Some of the elements of the cytoplasm begin to disintegrate, as does the lipid layer surrounding the fiber. Within a few days, the fiber has broken up into segments, taking on a ''beaded'' appearance in longitudinal sections. Eventually, the components of the degenerating fiber will disappear completely, the resulting void being filled by a redistribution of surrounding tissue, by a proliferation of glial cells, or, simply, by cerebrospinal fluid.

Another type of degenerative process, called **secondary degeneration,** occurs in the cell body as a result of transection of the axon. In many cases, particularly if the damage is inflicted close to the cell body, the neuron will die and disintegrate much like the distal portion of the fiber. But if the damage is somewhat further distant, the degenerative process may be reversible. Typically, there is a rearrangement of some of the cytoplasmic inclusions (e.g., the nucleus may adopt an eccentric position), and the Nissl substance of the cell may fade or temporarily disappear (chromatolysis). Then, after a period of days or weeks, these degenerative signs will begin to reverse, and the cell may once again appear to be normal. It should, of course, be emphasized that there is no evidence of complete functional recovery in the central nervous system; the distal portion of the fiber does not regenerate to its original terminals, although some sprouting of other fibers may take place (cf. Raisman, 1969).

A third type of degeneration, called **transneuronal degeneration,** is less easily understood (cf. Nauta & Ebbesson, 1970, Chapter 11). In cases in which large numbers of fibers undergo degeneration, it is not uncommon for the postsynaptic cells (which were not directly damaged) to undergo degeneration. Thus, the degenerative process crosses the synaptic barrier despite the fact that most evidence indicates that successive neurons are metabolically independent.

These degenerative processes can be observed to a certain extent with standard staining procedures (e.g., the cresylviolet stain is useful in detecting the changes in the appearance of the Nissl substance during secondary degeneration), but the most useful procedures have taken advantage of the fact that degenerating fibers are selectively impregnated by certain staining procedures. In 1904, Bielschowski found that cells in the process of degenerating were stained more heavily than normal fibers with the silver-staining techniques. This procedure was greatly improved by Nauta and Gygax (1954) and Nauta (1957), who developed procedures for suppressing the degree of impregnation of normal fibers by treatment with potassium permanganate. (The reasons for this effect are not fully understood.) When properly done, the cells and normal fibers are golden brown in appearance, while the degenerating fibers are dark brown or black. The use of this technique is somewhat tedious, but the results provide information that is simply unattainable through other staining procedures (cf. Nauta & Ebbesson, 1970, Chapters 5 and 6). A typical experiment utilizing this technique would be conducted as follows:

1. Surgical Damage. The first step is to produce damage to the fiber system that is being studied. This can be done by using a variety of techniques, including surgical aspiration, electrolytic lesions, or the transection of fiber bundles. Regardless of the procedure, the result, of course, is that the fibers that were damaged will begin to show degenerative processes.

2. Survival Time. One of the most critical variables is the period of survival of the animal after the damage has been produced. If the organism is sacrificed too soon follow-ing the damage, the staining properties of the damaged fibers will not differ significantly from those of normal fibers; if the organism is allowed to survive too long, the damaged fibers will have disintegrated and there will be no substrate for the stain. Thus, there is an optimal survival time which must be considered for this procedure. Unfortunately, there is no single survival time that applies to all systems. The time course of degeneration varies as a function of the size of the fibers, so different systems will have different optimal survival times. Moreover, to the extent that fiber diameter differs within the same system, varied survival times must be used to detect these different components of the system. Additionally, the temperature of the system during degeneration is an important variable that must be considered, especially with respect to poikilothermic animals. Because of these variables, the only recourse of the anatomist is to systematically vary the survival time and go through the tedious staining procedure for each one to determine the pattern of degeneration associated with surgical destruction that was produced. In the case of rodent brains, typical survival times are in the range of 2–14 days.

3. Suppression Time. As in any staining procedure, the timing of the various steps is critical. In the case of the degeneration stains, the step involving the suppression of the staining of normal fibers must be systematically varied for the best differentiation between normal and degenerating fibers to be determined. Usually, this is done by processing several sections from a particular brain and briefly examining the results. Based on this survey, the remaining sections are stained using two or three different suppression times in the range that is likely to be most effective. For example, if suppression times of 5, 10, 15, and 20 minutes indicate that 10 minutes is best, the remaining sections may be stained using suppression times of 7, 10, and 12 minutes. As in the case of the different survival times, there is no ''correct'' suppression time—it varies for different systems and for different aspects of the same system.

4. Evaluation. The most difficult aspect of the entire procedure is the microscopic evaluation of the stained tissue to determine the projection pathways of the damaged fibers. In theory, it should be a simple matter to trace the darkly stained fibers to their terminations. In practice, there are numerous pitfalls. Obviously, the survival time of the organism and the suppression time used during staining will change the appearance of the stained material. The major difficulty, however, lies in the possibility of artifacts. Even with the precautions of filtering all solutions, using triple-distilled water, and scrupulously attending to cleanliness of glassware, there will be some artifactual deposits of silver. In some cases, these aberrant stains will be deposited on the surface of the sections and can be recognized by carefully focusing through the depth of the section under high magnification—but it can still be troublesome. Less easy to recognize are the systems that, for reasons which remain mysterious, simply stain more darkly than other regions. One of the procedures for discriminating these normal fibers from degenerating fibers is to look carefully for the beaded appearance of the fibers that are in the process of degenera-tion. Even this can be difficult if the fibers are small in diameter or if, for some reason, the normal fibers are ''wavy'' and travel in and out of the plane of focus. The latter problem can usually be detected by carefully focusing through the section.

The problems inherent in this technique become even more complex when an attempt is made to follow the degenerating fibers all the way to the terminal boutons and to determine the nature of the synapse. The early staining procedures developed by Bielschow-ski (1904) and later by Nauta (1957) did not effectively stain these small-diameter processes of the axon. More recently, modifications by Fink and Heimer (1967) and de Olmos (1972) have resulted in considerable progress in staining these regions, although problems of interpretation remain.

In conclusion, the silver-staining procedures for degenerating fibers have been extremely useful in determining the interconnections of the central nervous system, but they have also tested the skill and patience of the neuroanatomists. The vagaries of survival time, suppression times, and artifacts are such that an anatomist is never willing to state flatly whether or not a dark-staining set of fibers represents degeneration. The accurate determination of the projections of a particular fiber bundle can be accomplished only by viewing a large number of sections in which the parameters of the staining procedure have been varied as well as sections that have been treated with different staining procedures. Even then, the cautious neuroanatomist will not be satisfied until the material has been studied by both light and electron microscopy. The reader who is especially interested in the techniques and problems in this area is referred to an excellent collection of papers in Nauta and Ebbesson's (1970) *Contemporary Research Techniques in Neuroanatomy* (see especially articles by Guillery, Chapter 5; Heimer, Chapter 8; and Ebbesson, Chapter 7).

HISTOCHEMICAL METHODS

Chemically Specific Stains

A number of stains have been developed during recent years that allow anatomists to selectively stain fibers that share certain chemical characteristics related to the neurotransmitter substance that is thought to be involved. One of the earliest and most successful attempts in this area was that of a group of Danish investigators (cf. Falck, 1962; Falck, Hillarp, Theme, & Torp, 1962). The basic procedure involves freeze-drying the fresh tissue and exposing it to formaldehyde vapors under specific conditions. The formaldehyde vapors form fluorescent chemical complexes with certain **biogenic amines** (e.g., dopamine, norepinephrine, and serotonin) that are believed to be neurotransmitters. When treated tissue is exposed to ultraviolet radiation under a fluorescent microscope, the complexes produce a shift in the wavelength of the light, causing fluorescence in the yellow and green range of the visible spectrum. These procedures, and later modifications, have been extremely useful in determining the location of neurons that contain these compounds. (See Fuxe, Hökfelt, Jonsson, & Ungerstedt, 1970, and Ungerstedt, 1971, for excellent reviews of these procedures.)

Another type of staining procedure has been used to identify fiber systems involving **acetylcholine** as a transmitter (cf. Shute & Lewis, 1963; Shute, 1972). The simplest procedure involves a logical jump that not all researchers are willing to make. The procedure selectively stains fibers that contain the enzyme acetylcholinesterase (AChE), which is involved in the degradation of acetylcholine. The rationale is that this specific enzyme would not be present unless its substrate, acetylcholine, was also present. This reasoning is somewhat risky in view of our limited knowledge of central nervous system pharmacology, but more recent procedures that allow the staining of the enzyme of synthesis, choline acetylase, have generally verified the results of the earlier experiments (cf. Lewis, Shute, & Silver, 1967). In this case, the logic is much tighter, and there is every reason to believe that these fibers contain acetylcholine as the neurotransmitter. Although it would be ideal to stain specifically for the putative neurotransmitter, the labile nature of acetylcholine has made this technically difficult.

Axoplasmic Transport Methods

Several procedures have been developed recently to take advantage of the fact that chemicals in the cell body of a neuron are transported down the axon to the terminal regions of the fiber. One of these procedures involves the injection of labeled amino acids into localized regions of the brain (see Cowan, Gottlieb, Hendrickson, Price, & Woolsey, 1972). The cells in that region take up the amino acids and incorporate them into cellular proteins that are then transported throughout the cell body and axon. The localization of the radioactivity, determined at various times after the injection, can give an indication of both the rate of axonal flow and the projection pathways of the fibers arising from the area of amino acid injection.

Another method that is technically simpler and has some additional advantages over the autoradiographic technique is the horseradish peroxidase procedure (see Lynch, Gall, Mensah, & Cotman, 1974). In this procedure, a small amount of horseradish peroxidase is injected into a restricted region of the brain. The cells take up the enzyme, and it is carried to the terminal regions via axonal transport mechanisms. The optimal survival time for this method is about three days after injection, at which time the frozen brain sections are stained via a procedure that is chemically specific for the enzyme horseradish peroxidase.

Other chemically specific stains have also been developed and will continue to be developed. To the extent that fibers that utilize a particular transmitter substance are involved in similar functions, these procedures may help to provide an important adjunct to the arsenal of stains outlined herein. Even if there is no similarity of function, the stains would be useful. In general, any staining procedure that allows one to *selectively* stain certain parts of the central nervous system—whether it be fibers, cell bodies, degenerating tissue, or enzyme systems—will provide an alternative way of viewing the structure of the brain. Eventually, the comparison of the results of all of these selective procedures will allow anatomists to describe the connections and functions of the central nervous system in much greater detail.

Electrophysiological Methods

Although most of the details of anatomical pathways have been based on studies using histological methods, important contributions have also been made with electrophysiological techniques. The interpretation of the electrophysiological data is somewhat more tenuous, being based on the recording of transient electrical signals rather than on the observation of physical structures. Yet, as it has been emphasized in the preceding sections, even the observations of the structures of the nervous system can be interpreted in a variety of ways depending upon the type of staining procedure that is used. Given the sometimes imprecise nature of the histological evidence and the fact that the electrophysiological procedures are usually more convenient and based on the functions of the nervous system, it is important to provide a brief summary of the rationale of these techniques.

The electrophysiological procedures rely on certain highly predictable functional aspects of neural tissue. These relationships have been studied intensively in the peripheral nervous system and with *in vitro* preparations of dissected nerves. Although the substructure of the brain is far too complicated to allow direct observations, the principles derived from these simple preparations allow inferences to be made with respect to the nature of the pathways that are being studied in the brain.

The basic procedure used in most studies entails the implantation of a stimulating electrode into one portion of the brain and a recording electrode at a somewhat distant site. The recording electrode can be designed to record either from a single cell (unit recordings) or from a population of cells. In either case, there will exist some background level of activity that reflects the normal, ongoing functions of the brain. The inference that neural pathways exist between the stimulating site and the recording site depends upon the recording of electrical events that are highly correlated in time with the delivery of impulses through the stimulating electrode.

Owing to the complexities of both anatomy and function, the relationships between the signals that are delivered and those that are recorded are usually rather complicated. But it is precisely these complications that provide evidence for the existence of certain types of pathways. A full explanation of functional characteristics of neurons is not necessary (see Brazier, 1961, and Ruch, Patton, Woodbury, & Towe, 1961, for more details), but the basic principles will be outlined.

Perhaps the most important characteristic of the neuron for these purposes is the fact that conduction velocity of the action potential is closely related to fiber diameter. In the case of myelinated axons, the conduction velocity is directly and linearly related to the diameter of the axon. For unmyelinated fibers, the conduction velocity is proportional to the square root of the fiber diameter. Since the distance between the stimulating and recording electrodes is known, the diameter of the fibers that course between the two locations can be estimated by determining the time between the delivery of a stimulus and the arrival of the onset of the response to that stimulus. Additional information can be derived by determining the threshold for effective stimulation—the amount of current required to stimulate a fiber being directly related to fiber size. Thus, it is possible to infer the presence of two or more populations of fibers based on the combination of effective stimulation intensities and the calculated conduction velocities.

In most cases, the relationships become more complicated due to the presence of the one or more synapses interposed between the stimulating and recording sites. The synapse imposes a delay of approximately 0.5 millisecond on the transmission of the action potential. Although this is a relatively short period of time, in many cases the delay cannot be accounted for by any other factors and can serve to verify the presence of one or more synapses. In these cases, the electrophysiological recordings may be more informative than histological procedures, which do not always successfully locate synaptic junctions.

In still more complicated preparations, it can be demonstrated that the production of action potentials is dependent upon the specific frequency of stimulation. The combination of the synaptic delays and the individual refractory periods of neurons can combine in such a way that stimulus frequencies above or below some critical frequency are ineffective in setting up electrical activity in a neuronal network. It should be emphasized that the number of variables that can account for these observations make it virtually impossible to unequivocally account for these higher order interactions. Under these circumstances, the electrophysiological procedures can do little more than determine that some multisynaptic pathway exists between the stimulating and recording sites.

Some recent research has utilized a combination of electrophysiological techniques and electron microscopy that may be particularly powerful in determining brain circuitry (see van Harreveld & Fifkova, 1975). The procedure combines the phenomenon of post-tetanic potentiation with a somewhat tedious procedure (freeze-substitution) for preparing the tissue for electron-microscopic examination. Post-tetanic potentiation refers to the observation that the delivery of a train of stimuli can reduce the threshold for subsequent stimulation. These investigators used square-wave pulses and delivered 30 sec of 30/sec stimulation (i.e., 900 stimuli) to the entorhinal cortex. Following stimulation, they removed the brain, sliced through the region of the hippocampus, and quickly placed the cut end of the block of tissue against a silver plug that was immersed in liquid nitrogen ($-206°C$). This procedure allows the thin layer of tissue immediately adjacent to the silver plug to be prepared for electron-microscopic examination. Careful inspection of these preparations revealed that the area of the dendritic spines (i.e., synaptic zones) was significantly greater for animals that had received stimulation than for control animals that did not receive the 900 stimuli. This is strong evidence that the appearance of the synaptic zone can be altered by stimulation and may provide a very powerful technique for the identification of neural circuits.

SUMMARY OF ANATOMICAL TERMS

Terms Defining Spatial Relationships (See Fig. 2–1)

The spatial relationships of the structures of the brain and other organs are defined by two major axes:

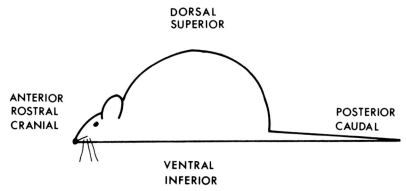

Fig. 2-1. Schematic summary of the terminology used to describe spatial relationships.

The longitudinal axis (nose-to-tail) is described in terms of **anterior** or **rostral** direction (toward the nose) and the **posterior** or **caudal** direction (toward the tail). The term **cranial** is also used occasionally to denote the anterior direction.

The transverse axis (belly-to-spine) is described in terms of the **ventral** or **inferior** direction (toward the belly surface) and the **dorsal** or **superior** direction (away from the belly surface).

Terms Defining Planes of Sections (See Fig. 2–2)

The planes just defined are also used to obtain more or less standard orientations when thin sections of brain tissue are examined. The planes of these sections are defined as follows:

The **coronal** plane consists of a vertical plane that passes through the brain perpendicular to the long axis. It is analogous to the slices in a loaf of bread.

The **horizontal** plane, as the name implies, consists of a horizontal or flat plane that passes through the brain parallel with the longitudinal axis. The blade of a rotary lawn mower travels in a horizontal plane.

The **sagittal** plane consists of a vertical plane that passes through the brain along the longitudinal axis. If the head is split down the midline, the resulting section is referred to as **midsagittal;** parallel sections that are displaced laterally from the midline are referred to as **parasagittal.**

Long slender structures, such as the spinal cord, may be cut in **cross section** or in **longitudinal** sections. By analogy, carrot slices are cross sections and carrot sticks are longitudinal sections.

Terms Defining Lateral Positions (See Fig. 2–3)

The central nervous system is bilaterally symmetrical and a number of terms are in common usage to denote relationships between the two sides:

The term **ipsilateral** refers to a structure that is on the same side. The left foot is ipsilateral to the left hand.

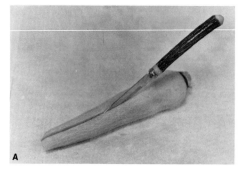
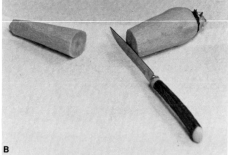

Fig. 2-2. Panel A uses a carrot to depict longitudinal sections. Panel B shows a cross section.

The term **contralateral** refers to a structure that is on the opposite side. The right hand is contralateral to both the left foot and the left hand.

The same structure on the opposite side is said to be in a **homotopic** position. The right hand is homotopic to the left hand, and the lateral amygdaloid nucleus is homotopic to the same nucleus on the opposite side. This term is not to be confused with the term **topographic,** which also denotes a point-to-point relationship, but with respect to two different structures. As an example, adjacent points on the retina project topographically to adjacent points on the visual cortex.

If a manipulation is performed on only one side, it is said to be a **unilateral** treatment; if performed on both sides, it is a **bilateral** treatment.

Terms Defining Units of the Nervous System

A single nerve cell is called a **neuron.** The long process that conducts the impulse away from the cell body of the neuron is called an **axon.**

A bundle of axons in the peripheral nervous system is called a **nerve;** a bundle of axons in the central nervous system is referred to as a **tract.** The visual system offers an interesting example in which the very same axons that form the optic nerve are termed the "optic tract" upon entry into the central nervous system proper. Smaller bundles of fibers in the brain are frequently termed **stria** or **fascicles.**

An aggregate of cell bodies in the peripheral nervous system is called a **ganglion.** A similar aggregate in the central nervous system is called a **nucleus.** A nucleus that is imbedded in a central fiber bundle is sometimes referred to as the **bed nucleus** of that bundle (e.g., the bed nucleus of the stria terminalis).

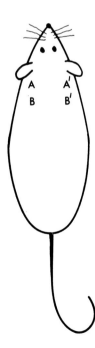

Fig. 2-3. Schematic summary of terms used to describe relative positions of structures. Locus A is said to be **ipsilateral** to locus B. Locus A is **contralateral** to both A′ and B′, but locus A′ is said to be a **homotopic** structure with respect to locus A.

Terms Defining Pathways of Fibers and Impulses (See Fig. 2–4)

Normally, the nerve impulse or action potential travels in only one direction—from the cell body to the end of the axon. This is termed the **orthodromic** direction. This results from the fact that the impulse arises from the region of the cell body. Under conditions of artificial stimulation, an impulse may be generated from a central portion of the axon. This impulse will travel in both the orthodromic direction and in the opposite, or **antidromic,** direction.

The transection of an axon along its central portion can lead to two types of degeneration of the remaining tissue. The degeneration that proceeds toward the end of the axon is termed **anterograde** degeneration; degeneration of the tissue back toward the cell body is termed **retrograde** degeneration.

The brain communicates with the remainder of the body by two major categories of nerve fibers: **Afferent** fibers carry information into or toward the brain; **efferent** fibers carry impulses away from the brain. Within the central nervous system the suffixes -**fugal**

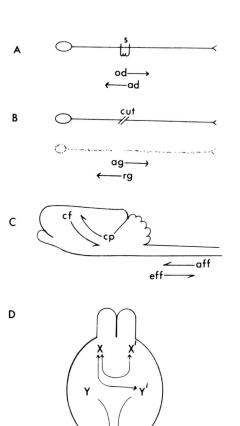

Fig. 2-4. Summary of terminology used to indicate the directions of events. In panel A, the delivery of a stimulus (s) to an axon can result in the propagation of an action potential in both the orthodromic (od) direction and the antidromic (ad) direction. In panel B, the transection (cut) of a fiber always results in anterograde (ag) degeneration and can also lead to retrograde (rg) degeneration including the cell body. In panel C, it is shown that afferent (aff) fibers travel toward the brain, whereas efferent (eff) fibers travel away from the brain; within the brain, fibers that travel toward the cortex are corticopetal (cp), whereas fibers that leave the cortex are termed corticofugal (cf). In panel D, the connections between homotopic regions such as X and X′ are termed **commissures;** connections between contralateral regions are termed **crossed projections** (e.g., X to Y′); the crossing of long pathways en route to the termination (e.g., Y and Y′ to Z and Z′) is referred to as a **decussation.**

and -**petal** are sometimes used to denote fibers that travel away from or toward a particular location, respectively. For example, fibers traveling toward the cortex are cortico**petal,** whereas fibers that are leaving the cortex are cortico**fugal.**

Owing to the bilateral symmetry of the nervous system, there are numerous instances in which fibers cross from one side to the other. There are several terms used to denote these crossings, and there is sometimes confusion as to the precise meanings of these terms. The term **commissure** refers to the crossing of fibers that are connecting a particular structure on one side of the brain with the homotopic structure on the other side. Pathways that project to a different structure on the contralateral side are, technically, **crossed projections.** As indicated in the discussion of the olfactory system (cf. Chapter 9), recent anatomical findings have revealed that the anterior commissure is actually a crossed projection. The term **decussation** is used to describe the point of crossing of two long fiber bundles (e.g., the pyramidal tracts). The term **chiasm** also refers to this type of crossing but is used almost exclusively for the fibers of the optic system.

The Limbic System Defined   3

INTRODUCTION

The term "limbic system," coined in 1952 by MacLean, represents over three centuries of changing conceptual boundaries and terminology concerning a group of brain structures. The reasons for this continuing controversy are attributable to the different ways in which a set of structures can be organized conceptually. One method is simply to name each identifiable structure in the brain with no attempt to consolidate the individual units into groups. While this procedure has the advantage of eliminating controversy as to the appropriate subdivisions, the result would be chaotic. Even if there is not total agreement, general categories, such as hydrocarbons, mammals, and perhaps even the limbic system, can serve as useful concepts within their respective fields of science.

A second method is to group the individual structures on the basis of function. This is possibly the most attractive scheme of organization, but, unfortunately, the function of many of the structures is not known in any detail, a situation which leads to considerable speculation and disagreement. Many of the structures that are currently included as parts of the limbic system have been termed the **rhinencephalon** in reference to the presumed olfactory function of these structures. As explained by White (1970), the term had been used in literary works but was first used as a term denoting a portion of the brain by Owen in 1868. Owen restricted the term to include only the olfactory bulb and the olfactory peduncle, but Turner (1890) included the pyriform lobe in his definition of the term.

A third method is to group individual structures on the basis of their evolutionary development and the detailed cellular organization of the structures. Elliot Smith (1896, 1910) used such a scheme to establish three major subdivisions that signified the phylogenetic development of the **pallium,** or outer layer of the brain. The oldest cortical structures were termed the **archipallium,** which consisted primarily of the hippocampus. The somewhat more recent structures of the basal cortex (primarily the pyriform lobe) were termed the **paleocortex.** The remaining, most recently developed aspects of the cortical mantle were termed the **neopallium,** or neocortex (see Fig. 3–1).

A fourth method of categorization is to group the structures on the basis of their

25

location with respect to other structures. The earliest groupings of the structures now included in the limbic system were made according to this criterion. White (1970) has reviewed the historical development of this nomenclature and points out that Willis referred to this region of the brain as a **limbus,** or border, as early as 1664. The same region was later referred to as the **circonvolution de l'ourlet** (Foville, 1844) and as the **falciform lobe** (Schwalbe, 1881). The term which gained most widespread acceptance was Broca's (1878) **le grand lobe limbique,** which has been Anglicized into the **limbic lobe.**

The term **limbic system,** as defined by MacLean (1952), is based on a combination of criteria. The structures include those that were first described by Broca on the basis of location and spatial orientation. Some additional structures have been added because of similarities in function and the demonstration of anatomical connections (cf. Papez, 1937; Nauta, 1958). More recently, the same criteria have led Nauta and others to add still more structures so that the limbic system now encompasses structures in the midbrain, the hypothalamus, and even the neocortex (cf. Nauta, 1958; Powell, 1973). In most cases, the individual structures that are included in this classification have been carefully defined and disagreement is usually based on the inclusion or exclusion of the structure rather than on the precise boundaries of the structure. Thus, the grouping of these structures into a system simply provides a useful framework upon which research and speculation can be based. The framework can be changed, if required, by the addition of new data or by more meaningful theoretical expositions. It is this expanded and flexible use of the term ''limbic system'' that is used in this text.

Before proceeding to a discussion of the relationship of the limbic system to other portions of the brain, it should be pointed out that several of the major structures have a

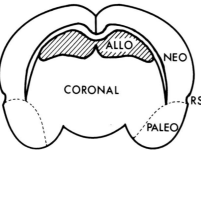

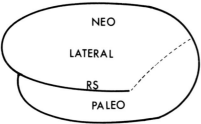

Fig. 3-1. Coronal and lateral views showing the allocortical (ALLO), paleocortical (PALEO), and neocortical (NEO) divisions of the rat brain. RS = rhinal sulcus.

long history of aliases. These aliases usually reflect the imagination of the anatomist in comparing the shape of the structure with some more common object. For example, the term **hippocampus** was first introduced by Arantius in 1587 because of a presumed similarity of the structure to a sea horse. As an alternative, Arantius suggested the term **Bombyx** to denote the similarity to a silkworm. Since that time, according to Tilney (1938), this structure has looked like ram's horns (**cornu arietis; cornu Ammonis**), like feet (**pes hippocampi**), like bird claws (**calcar avis**), and even like a hippopotamus (**pes hippopotami**). Likewise, the **septum** has been referred to as the **paraolfactory area,** the **paraterminal body of Elliot Smith,** and the **telencephalon impar** (see White, 1970). Even though most of this archaic terminology has been abandoned, the official nomenclature of the subdivisions of the septum is the **nucleus lateralis septi, nucleus medialis septi, nucleus triangularis septi, nucleus accumbens septi,** and **nucleus septofimbrialis.** These terms are awkward to use, especially for students who are just entering the bewildering field of neuroanatomy. In a letter to *Science,* Riggs (1975) emphasized the importance of maintaining common names by quoting the following passage by Wald (1952):

> In the original version of this table, Nuttal mentions *Cynocephalus mormon* and *sphinx,* omitting their common names. I have learned since that one is the mandrill, the other the guinea baboon. Since Nuttal wrote in 1904, these names have undergone the following vagaries. *Cynocephalus mormon* became *Papio mormon,* otherwise *Papio maimon,* which turned to *Papio sphinx.* This might well have been confused with *Cynocephalus,* now become *Papio sphinx,* had not the latter meanwhile been turned into *Papio papio.* This danger averted, *Papio sphinx* now became *Mandrillus sphinx,* while *Papio papio* became *Papio comatus.* All I can say to this is, thank heavens one is called the mandrill, the other the guinea baboon. (p. 399)

To the extent that it is possible, this text will use terms such as "mandrill" and "guinea baboon" in defining the structures and interconnections of the limbic system.

ONTOGENETIC AND PHYLOGENETIC DEVELOPMENT

The nervous system can be conceptualized as being composed of three neurons: an afferent neuron, an interneuron, and an efferent neuron. In primitive organisms, there may be relatively few of each type of neuron, but as the organism becomes increasingly complex, the number of sensory and motor neurons shows a proportionate increase, while the population of interneurons shows a *disproportionately* large increase. This relative increase in the size of the brain appears to represent the development and qualitative reorganization of various subsystems rather than a simple expansion of cell numbers. A comparison of primitive species with more recent species in terms of brain development and behavior may help to provide additional clues to the functions of the developing systems.

Phylogeny

Although the fossil record of brain tissue is very sparse, data from skull structure and from the study of the brains of existing species can provide some information regarding the phylogenetic development of the brain. For this purpose a few levels of development will be outlined.

One of the most primitive brains in our ancestral linkage is that of the cyclostome, a primitive fish (cf. Sarnat & Netsky, 1974). The forebrain of this species is comprised of a relatively thin layer of tissue on either side of the ventricle (see Fig. 3–2). The regions that are thought to be homologous to the hippocampus, pyriform cortex, corpus striatum, and septum of higher species are indicated. A similar arrangement exists for more advanced species of fish (e.g., Crossopterygia), the major difference being a thickening of the forebrain mantle.

In the amphibian brain, the forebrain structures have completely surrounded the ventricle, with the hippocampus and septum occupying the medial surface and the pyriform cortex and corpus striatum on the outer surface. This arrangement continues into the reptilian brain, the major difference being an enlargement of the corpus striatum into the lateral aspect of the ventricle and the first appearance of a small slip of neocortical tissue.

There appear to be at least two major lines of evolution from the primitive reptilian ancestry: one for birds and one for mammals. Precise homology of related areas is especially difficult, but the available evidence suggests that neocortical cells from the region of the **dorsal ventricular ridge** have migrated medially into the corpus striatum of birds and laterally in mammals to form a cortical mantle. In the latter case, there has been a progressive expansion of the neocortical mantle until it forms a thick layer over virtually the entire forebrain of higher species.

The rapid expansion of the neocortex in mammalian evolution has made it difficult to assess the rate of development of limbic system structures. Many investigators have compared the size of limbic structures with the size of the entire brain, concluding that most of these structures have regressed in higher mammalian forms, especially in man. More recently, Andy and Stephan (1968) have argued forcefully against this approach, suggesting that the comparisons should be made against relatively static systems, such as the brain stem, the spinal cord, or body size. Using these indices, which eliminate the influence of the rapidly expanding neocortex, there is a progressive increase in the size of the septal nuclei, with the peak of development being reached in man. If this argument is correct, it can be concluded that both the limbic system structures and the neocortex have expanded during mammalian evolution, with the expansion of the latter being much more dramatic.

Ontogeny

The central nervous system begins as a groove in the ectoderm of the embryo, develops into a hollow tube, then becomes increasingly larger and more complex until the adult form can be seen as a myriad of interconnections between billions of cells (see Fig. 3–3). Despite the complexity of this system, there is a high degree of order—the development proceeds in a highly systematic fashion with the final result being a virtually identical set of nuclei and fiber connections for all members of the same species. Although there are slight differences in the appearance of the various brain regions (just as there are differences in the appearance of faces, although all are basically the same), the similarities

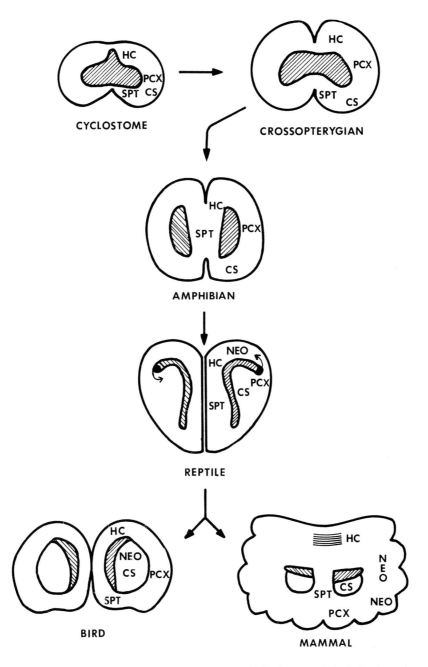

Fig. 3-2. This highly schematized summary of the phylogenetic development of the brain shows the major changes that have taken place in the forebrain. The primitive cyclostome shows a relatively undifferentiated wall of tissue around the ventricle. This wall of tissue thickens somewhat in amphioxus and comes to surround the ventricle in amphibians. Both the mass and the structural complexity are increased in reptiles, with the boundaries of the hippocampus (HC), septum (SPT), corpus striatum (CS), and pyriform cortex (PCX) becoming more distinct. Additionally, the first indication of neocortical tissue (NEO) is seen on the dorsal ventricular ridge. This new type of tissue appears to take two separate lines of development. In birds, it migrates ventrally and becomes incorporated into the so-called neostriatum. In mammals, it migrates dorsally and expands into the neocortical mantle.

are much more striking. If this were not the case, there could be no study of neuroanatomy.

As in the case of other systems, the ontogenetic development of the central nervous system is roughly parallel to the course of phylogenetic development; the early embryonic stages of advanced organisms resemble the embryonic stages of more primitive organisms. In general, this leads to a caudal-to-rostral sequence of development that has been termed **encephalization.** The neural substrates for the spinal reflexes and the reflex control systems of the brain stem are the first to develop. More anterior regions of the brain progress more slowly.

One of the most consistent measures of the progress of development is the extent of myelinization of fibers. In the peripheral nervous system, this insulating lipid layer is formed by Schwann cells; in the central nervous system it is formed by oligodendrocytes, specialized glial cells that may contain up to 70% of the cholesterol content of the brain. In the rat, the process of myelinization first begins in the spinal nerves and is completed by about 2 days after birth. The process is completed at progressively later ages for the spinal cord and cranial nerves (7 days postnatally), brain stem and thalamus (10–12 days postnatally), and cortex (14–26 days postnatally). Actually, the process is not completed in the latter two regions until the rat is 40–180 days of age (i.e., well into adulthood).

The presence of myelin is important for the functioning of the nervous system, its presence producing a several-fold increase in the conduction velocity of fibers. It is clear from the developmental timetable that the forebrain structures of the limbic system do not reach functional maturity until the rat is at least several weeks old. Accordingly, an assessment of behavioral capacities as a function of age may indicate the functional importance of these systems.

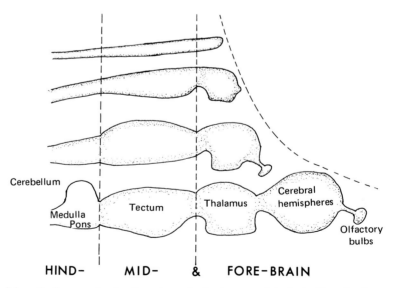

Fig. 3-3. Schematic diagrams showing the ontogenetic development of the brain. Note the disproportionate expansion of the forebrain relative to the midbrain and hindbrain.

Another useful index of development is the structure of the cells that make up the various nuclear regions. Although the total number of cells that will make up the brain has already been established at birth, these cells show considerable growth after the time of birth (i.e., the number of cells remains constant, but there is a large increase in the number of synaptic connections). An example of this type of development is the growth of long apical dendrites that typify cortical tissue. These dendrites become increasingly larger and more complex as a function of age and do not reach their peak size for at least several weeks in the rat and until as much as 30 years in man. Altman and Das (1965) have found a rapid sixfold increase in the number of differentiated granule cells in the dentate gyrus of rats, this increase taking place between the ages of 10 and 25 days. (It should be pointed out that this varies with the general degree of development of the species at the time of birth. In such animals as the rat, mouse, rabbit, and man a great deal of development takes place after birth; in such animals as guinea pigs, cattle, sheep, and swine a greater degree of development is present at the time of birth.)

The combination of behavioral, histochemical, and pharmacological techniques has also provided insight into the timetable of development, albeit less directly than strict anatomical measures. Histochemical techniques have revealed that the limbic system is interconnected with the midbrain through at least three great longitudinal fiber systems: specifically, an adrenergic system concentrated primarily within the medial forebrain bundle, a cholinergic system that is apparently identical with the ascending reticular activating system, and a serotonergic system that originates in the midbrain raphe region and ascends into forebrain structures (see Chapter 11).

Campbell and associates (Campbell, Lytle, & Fibiger, 1969; Mabry & Campbell, 1974) have performed a series of studies, utilizing a combination of pharmacological and behavioral techniques, that showed different rates of development of these systems. The adrenergic system appears to be the first to reach functional maturity, since infant rats (10 days of age) respond to amphetamine injections in much the same way as do adults. The development of the cholinergic system occurs later, as evidenced by the fact that adult-like responses to scopolamine injections are observed at 25 days of age but not at 18 days or earlier. The development of the serotonergic system appears to progress at an intermediate rate, showing the most rapid rate of development between the rat ages of 10 and 15 days (cf. Williams *et al.*, 1975). Experiments from other laboratories have shown that these same behaviors are easily influenced by pharmacological or surgical manipulation of the limbic system. Taken together, these results suggest that the functional maturation of these major fiber systems is dependent upon the establishment of connections with limbic system structures.

Some Concluding Remarks

Although the limbic system is a relatively old phylogenetic development, it has expanded along with the neocortex. This set of structures is in no sense a closed system—quite the contrary, the limbic system stands interposed between the neocortex, the hypothalamic-pituitary axis, and the major sensory systems. This strategic anatomical location places the limbic system in a position to become involved in the wide variety of behavioral and physiological functions that have been outlined, but until recently, the level of involvement may have been underestimated because of a failure to appreciate the potential for interaction with the neocortex.

MacLean (1970) has presented a simple model of the evolution of the brain that may help in the understanding of the relationship of the limbic system to other regions of the brain. He has termed the brain stem, basal ganglia, and thalamic regions the **reptilian brain,** because of the virtual lack of cortical structures in reptiles. These regions of the brain control reflexive events and simple behaviors that are directly related to the survival of the organism. The brain becomes more complex in mammals with the addition of the relatively simple limbic cortex. MacLean refers to these additional structures that form a sort of cap around the reptilian brain as the **paleomammalian brain,** which corresponds to the limbic system. During the more recent periods of evolution, these structures have, in turn, been capped with a more complicated form of cortex termed the ''neocortex.'' MacLean refers to this cortical mantle as the **neomammalian brain.** The behavior of modern mammals that essentially have the paleomammalian brain is considerably more complicated than the behavior of reptiles, with indications that the organisms have the capability of modulating behavior more precisely in terms of the prevailing environmental conditions. The behavior of higher mammals that have neocortical structures is correspondingly more complex, so that the behavior of the organism at any given moment may be almost totally independent of the internal environment or certain aspects of the external environment. This freedom from the almost reflexive response to internal conditions (e.g., depletion of the energy stores) and the appropriate aspects of the external environment (e.g., the availability of food) allows the organism to survive in a much more complicated environment, in which predators, social influences, or other environmental restraints may have greater importance. Further consideration of the structural and functional aspects of the limbic system will be given in Chapter 12, with more detailed summaries of anatomical connections presented in Chapters 4–10.

General Topography of the Limbic System

4

INTRODUCTION

As indicated in the first chapter, the use of the term "rhinencephalon" diminished as it became apparent that the anatomical relationships of these structures with the olfactory system were less prominent than originally thought (Brodal, 1947). Although the initial tendency was to use Broca's terminology, "limbic lobe," more recent usage seems to favor the term "limbic system" (e.g., MacLean, 1952). This modern substitution of the term "system" instead of "lobe" is probably the result of the identification of numerous interconnections among the various structures. In fact, the identification of anatomical connections has been the basis for including several additional structures within the so-called limbic system. Although there is no universal agreement as to which structures are to be included in the limbic system, the structures most commonly included are the hippocampus, the cingulate gyrus, the septum, the amygdala, the entorhinal cortex, and parts of the hypothalamus and midbrain.

The purpose of this chapter is to present an overview of the limbic system and introduce the various planes of transection that will be used throughout the text. The development of a firm grasp of the three-dimensional characteristics of these structures at this time will greatly enhance the ability to learn the more detailed characteristics that will be described in later sections.

With the exception of the midbrain component, the structures of the limbic system can still be viewed as a ringlike set of structures, even though a number of structures have been added since Broca originally described them. Perhaps the easiest way to grasp the gross spatial relationships is to imagine that these structures make up various segments of two donuts that are angled together toward the front and joined at the midline. The anteromedial portion of these rings would be occupied by the septum and the anterior thalamus, the dorsal portions by the cingulate gyri, the posterior portions by the hippocampi, and the ventral portions by the amygdala and hypothalamus.

A somewhat more realistic, though still highly schematic, view is shown in Figure 4–1. As indicated by the diagram, the various structures of the limbic system are interconnected via some rather prominent bundles of fibers. For the present purposes, these fiber bundles will be discussed only in terms of their obvious gross anatomical relationships to the various large nuclear masses. It should be kept in mind, however, that the detailed origins and terminations of these fiber bundles are considerably more diverse than suggested either by the model shown in Figure 4–1 or by gross dissection of the brain. In fact, these fiber bundles will serve as focal points around which the various anatomical relationships will be outlined in succeeding chapters.

THE HIPPOCAMPUS

The most prominent and easily identified structure of the limbic system is the **hippocampus.** The early neuroanatomists were intrigued by the shape of this structure, which some thought resembled a sea horse—hence, the term **hippocampus.** Others thought that the structure was more like the rams' horns which characterized the statues of Ammon and termed the structure **cornu Ammonis,** or Ammon's horn. Although this latter term still appears occasionally, the term ''hippocampus'' is by far the most commonly used. This structure can be rather easily exposed in gross dissection by removal of the cortex, as indicated in Figure 4–2.

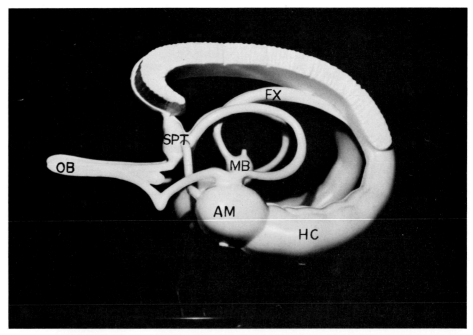

Fig. 4-1. Model of human limbic system (with permission of Hoffman-LaRoche Pharmaceutical Co.) based on a drawing by MacLean. Major structures include the hippocampus (HC), amygdala (AM), septum (SPT), mammillary bodies (MB), olfactory bulbs (OB), and fornix (FX).

The unique shape and relatively large size of the hippocampus make it an ideal structure for learning to combine the techniques of gross dissection and microscopic examination of histological material in order to gain an appreciation of the three-dimensional characteristics of a structure.

As shown in Figure 4–3, there are three commonly used planes of transection: (1) the **coronal,** or **frontal,** plane presents the structures in sections as they would be viewed from the front of the brain; (2) the **sagittal** plane presents structures in sections as they would be viewed from the side: if the section is made directly through the midline, it is termed a **midsagittal** section; if it is laterally displaced from the midline, it is termed a **parasagittal** section; (3) the **horizontal** plane presents structures in sections as they would be viewed from the top. With practice, it is relatively easy to translate a series of two-dimensional sections into a three-dimensional structure.

The first section of the hippocampus, illustrated in Figure 4–4, is a parasagittal section that was taken some distance from the midline. At this level, only the large, posterior portion of the hippocampus can be seen. Closer to the midline (Fig. 4–5), it can be seen that the anterior and dorsal aspects of the hippocampus become smaller in size and merge into a large bundle of fibers, the **fornix,** which interconnects the hippocampus with the **septum** and **hypothalamus.** The fornix fibers split to form (1) a compact post-commissural division (usually called the ''columns of the fornix'') which descends just posterior to the anterior commissure and (2) a more diffuse precommissural division that travels throughout the septal region.

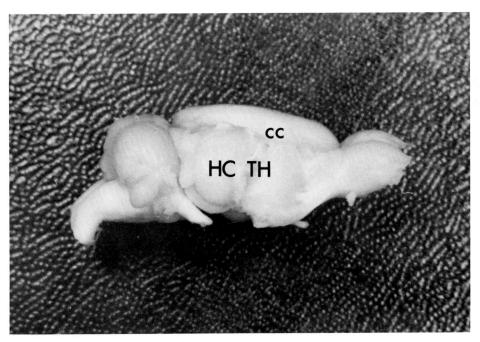

Fig. 4-2. The curved structure of the hippocampus (HC) can be easily seen in this dissection, in which the overlying cortex and the basal ganglia have been removed. The corpus callosum (CC) and the thalamus (TH) provide additional landmarks.

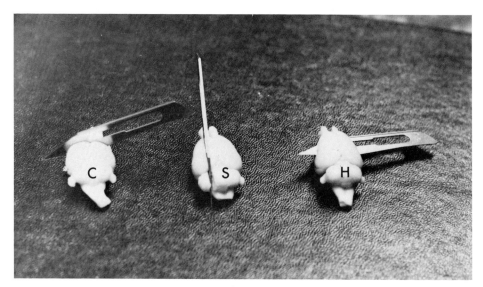

Fig. 4-3. The three most commonly used planes of transection are the coronal plane (C), the sagittal plane (S), and the horizontal plane (H).

The series of sections shown in Figure 4–6 shows the appearance of the hippocampus in coronal sections of the brain. The anterior-most aspect of the hippocampus is composed largely of the fibers of the fornix. In this plane, the fibers are seen in cross section, as in looking at the cut end of a rope. More posteriorly, there is still a large component of fibers, but the characteristic "jelly-roll" appearance of the hippocampus becomes appar-

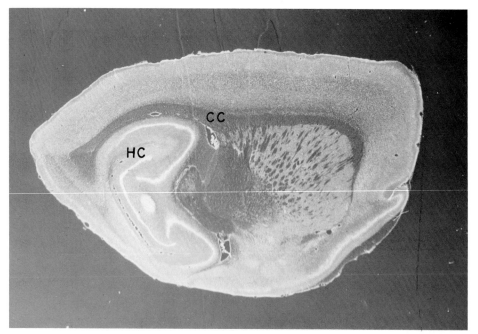

Fig. 4-4. Parasagittal section showing the large posterior portion of the hippocampus (HC). The corpus callosum (CC) is also indicated as a reference point.

ent. It should also be noted that the hippocampal structures diverge. Still more posteriorly, the hippocampus is seen in two locations—a dorsal component and a ventral component. The ventral component is the tip of the horn, which has curved downward and anteriorly into the temporal lobe region. Figure 4–6D shows a section through the hippocampus as it curves downward into the temporal lobe. As will be seen in a later chapter, the detailed structure of the hippocampus is rather complicated. These complications become downright tedious to follow due to the hornlike shape of the structure—in order to follow the structure in any sort of consistent manner, it would be necessary to make histological sections in a widely varying set of planes to maintain a ''cross-sectional'' view of the coiled jelly roll (see Fig. 4–7).

Technically speaking, the structure which is shown in dissection in Figure 4–4 should be termed the **hippocampal complex,** because the details of the structural variations suggest that it should be subdivided into several different components. For example, one subdivision of the complex is the **dentate gyrus,** which can be seen by comparing Figure 4–6(B,C,D) with Figure 5–2. Both the dentate gyrus and the hippocampus proper have been further subdivided into layers and subdivisions of these layers on the basis of the detailed anatomical characteristics of the individual cells. These cytoarchitectonic subdivisions will be considered in Chapter 5.

Another closely related structure is the **subiculum,** which occupies the region between the hippocampus proper and the entorhinal cortex. The term ''subiculum'' means cave and is derived from the shape of this band of tissue as it follows the arch of the posterior hippocampus. An easy way to visualize this structure is to imagine pressing the hippocampal complex into a mass of clay; the wall of the resulting cavelike depression would roughly correspond to the outline of the subiculum.

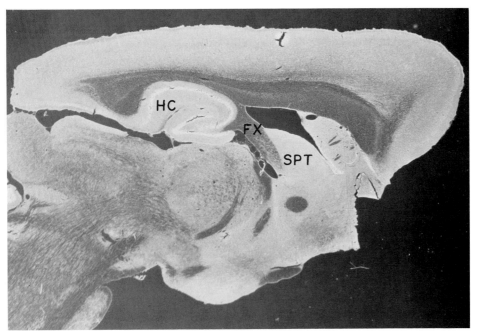

Fig. 4-5. Parasagittal section near the midline showing the more medial and dorsal aspects of the hippocampus (HC), along with the septum (SPT) and the fibers of the fornix (FX) that interconnect these structures.

As indicated in Figure 4–5, the anterior portion of the hippocampus becomes continuous with the fornix, which, in turn, courses into the septal region. The **septum** is composed of a group of nuclei and fibers which are nested beneath the broad band of fibers that make up the **corpus callosum** and between the lateral ventricles. The ventral border of the septum is somewhat less clearly defined but is approximately at the level of the **anterior commissure** (this fiber bundle will be described later). The series of coronal sections in Figure 4–8 show the relationship of the septal region to the structures noted previously as well as the nuclear subdivisions of the septum. In the most anterior regions of the septum, two thin bands of cells make up the **medial and lateral** septal nuclei. More posteriorly, the medial septal nucleus remains rather small amid the fibers and the nucleus of the **diagonal band.** By contrast, the lateral nuclei are more sparsely infiltrated with fibers and become very prominent bilateral structures. Near the posterior border of the septum, the fibers of the fornix columns descend through this structure and two additional septal nuclei become apparent—the **triangular nucleus** of the septum, which fills the small triangle formed between the fornix columns, and the **septofimbrial nuclei,** which are embedded within the fornix system. Closely associated with, but technically not a part of, the septum are the **bed nuclei** of the **stria terminalis** and the **anterior commissure.** In addition, there is the rather large **nucleus accumbens,** which in its complete nomenclature (nucleus accumbens septi), means the nucleus leaning against the septum.

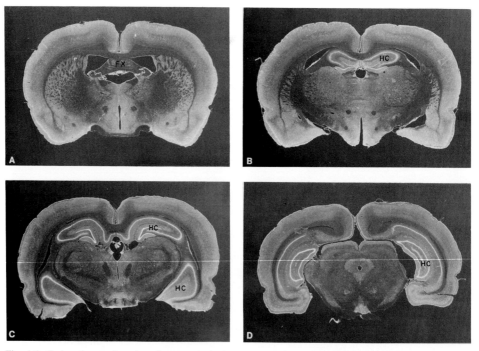

Fig. 4-6. Series of coronal sections from successively more posterior regions of the hippocampus (HC). Compare these figures with the appearance of different anteroposterior levels of Figures 4-4 and 4-5. The relatively compact bundle of fornix fibers (FX) represents the anterior-most regions of the hippocampal complex (panel A). More posterior sections (panels B and C) show the layered structure of both the dorsal and ventral portions of the hippocampus. Panel D shows a section through the large posterior portion of the hippocampus.

THE HYPOTHALAMUS

The ventral border of the septal region is continuous with the anterior portions of a set of nuclei and fibers that comprise the medial region of the base of the brain. These structures are known collectively as the **hypothalamus.** Several aspects of the hypothalamus can be observed on the ventral surface of the whole brain. As shown in Figure 4–9, the **optic nerves** converge and partially decussate to form the **optic chiasm,** which is attached at the base of the brain. Following this decussation, the fibers become a part of the central nervous system proper and are hence termed the **optic tracts.** Immediately posterior to the optic chiasm is the root of the **infundibulum,** from which the pituitary was torn off during the removal of the brain from the skull. The posterior border of the hypothalamus is marked by a conspicuous elevation called the **mammillary bodies** (this structure is present in larger mammals as a pair of protuberances—hence the name ''mammillary bodies''). These landmarks should be used as reference points for the major nuclear subdivisions of the hypothalamus that are shown in Figure 4–10.

The anterior border of the hypothalamus is in approximately the same plane as the most anterior parts of the anterior commissure and the optic chiasm. At this level, the cluster of cells surrounding the third ventricle represents the anterior portion of the **preoptic nucleus.** In addition to this **medial** portion of the preoptic nucleus, there is a more **lateral** subdivision which lies interposed between the fibers of the diagonal band and the medial forebrain bundle. Still further laterally, there is a small cluster of rather large cells that make up the **magnocellular** division of the preoptic nucleus. More posteriorly, the medial portion of the preoptic nucleus becomes quite prominent, while the more lateral divisions remain small.

There are two major landmarks which can be associated with the posterior border of the preoptic nucleus: (1) The postcommissural fornix columns have turned posteriorly and are, therefore, seen in cross section just dorsal to the hypothalamus; and (2) two small, darkly stained structures, the **suprachiasmatic nuclei,** are present on the dorsomedial surface of the optic chiasm. The lateral borders of the optic chiasm are marked by another pair of darkly stained structures, the **supraoptic nuclei.** At this level, virtually the entire medial aspect of the hypothalamus is occupied by the **anterior hypothalamic nucleus.** (A thin band of cells along the walls of the third ventricle constitute the **periventricular**

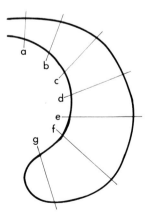

Fig. 4-7. The schematic diagram of the curved hippocampal structure depicts the difficulties that would be encountered in trying to maintain a ''cross-sectional'' view of the hippocampus. The various hypothetical planes (a–g) are indicated.

nucleus.) More laterally, the fibers of the medial forebrain bundle are interspersed with the cell bodies of the **lateral hypothalamic nucleus.**

The posterior edge of the optic chiasm (i.e., the point at which the optic tracts begin to diverge) serves as a landmark for a somewhat diffuse band of fibers which cross the ventral surface of the hypothalamus. These fibers are known as the **supraoptic commissure.** At this level, the postcommissural fornix columns have moved down into the hypothalamus proper, marking the dorsolateral borders of the now more compact anterior hypothalamic nuclei. The **paraventricular nuclei** form a mushroom-shaped structure surrounding the third ventricle. The lateral borders of this nucleus are typically stained rather darkly.

Moving still further posteriorly, the optic tracts are now seen more laterally and are interposed between the fibers of the **internal capsule** and the nuclei of the **amygdala.** The dorsal border of the hypothalamus is marked by a pair of wedge-shaped structures composed of fibers and cell bodies known as the **zona incerta.** The fornix fibers are now rather small and compact, lying on the medial aspect of the **medial forebrain bundle.** At this level, the **paraventricular nuclei** once again occupy only a thin band surrounding the ventricle. The ventral portion of the medial aspect of the hypothalamus is occupied by the **ventromedial nuclei** of the hypothalamus. Just dorsal to this pair of nuclei are the **dorsomedial nuclei** of the hypothalamus.

The most prominent structures in the posterior region of the hypothalamus form the

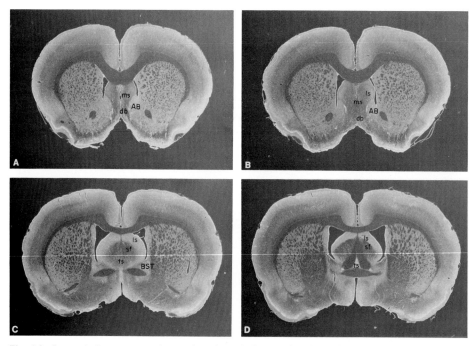

Fig. 4-8. Successively more posterior sections through the septal region. The medial portion of the septal complex is occupied by the medial septal nucleus (ms), the nucleus of the diagonal band (db), and the triangular nucleus of the septum (ts). More laterally, are the large lateral septal nuclei (ls) and the septofimbrial nuclei (sf). Closely related to the septal nuclei are the nucleus accumbens (AB) and the bed nucleus of the stria terminalis (BST).

mammillary complex. The various subdivisions of this structure form the entire base of the hypothalamus. At this level, the fornix bundle becomes rather sparse as it terminates in the mammillary bodies, and the fibers of the **mammillothalamic tract** can be seen in several bundles as they leave the mammillary bodies and course toward the anterior thalamic nuclei. The dorsal and medial aspect of the hypothalamus at this level is occupied by the **posterior nuclei** of the hypothalamus. The fibers of the **medial forebrain bundle,** which are no longer associated with the lateral hypothalamic nucleus, are located just dorsal to the lateral regions of the mammillary complex.

THE AMYGDALOID COMPLEX

The nuclei of the **amygdala** form an almond-shaped structure ("amygdala" means almond) which is nested between the inferomedial aspect of the cortex and the lateral border of the hypothalamus. The anterior-to-posterior extent of this nuclear mass is approximately the same as that of the hypothalamus. A convenient landmark for the anterior border of the amygdala is the appearance of the slitlike third ventricle; the posterior border coincides with the posterior extent of the mammillary complex.

The sections shown in Figure 4–11(A–D) indicate that the rather poorly demarcated **anterior amygdaloid area** merges almost imperceptibly into the hypothalamus at its

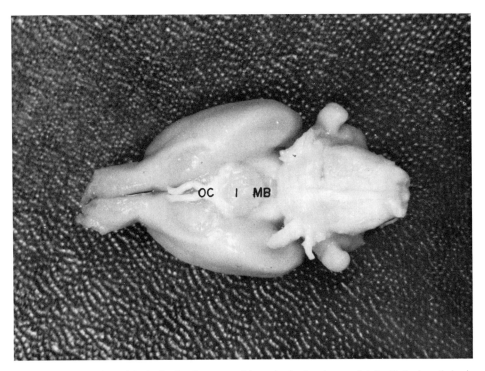

Fig. 4-9. Ventral surface of the brain showing some of the major landmarks associated with the hypothalamic region. The anterior border is marked by the optic chiasm (OC), the infundibulum (I) or stalk of the pituitary is in the central region, and the mammillary bodies (MB) comprise the posterior region.

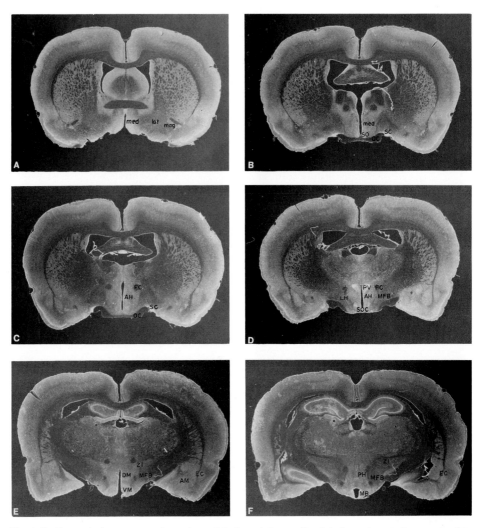

Fig. 4-10. Successively more posterior regions of the hypothalamus. Panel A shows the anterior aspects of the hypothalamus, including the medial (med), lateral (lat), and magnocellular (mag) divisions of the preoptic nucleus (PO). As shown in panel B, the medial preoptic nucleus becomes quite large in more posterior sections. Just posterior to the preoptic region (panel C), the hypothalamus is sandwiched just beneath the postcommissural fornix columns (FC) and just above the fibers of the optic chiasm (OC). Closely associated with the optic chiasm are the suprachiasmatic (SC) and supraoptic (SO) nuclei. Also shown are the periventricular nucleus (PV), the anterior nucleus (AH), and the medial forebrain bundle (MFB). Panel D shows a continuation of these same structures, along with the appearance of the supraoptic commissure (SOC). More posteriorly (panel E), several additional nuclei appear, including the dorsomedial (DM) and ventromedial (VM) hypothalamic nuclei. The fibers of the medial forebrain bundle (MFB) form relatively compact bundles at this level. Adjacent structures include the amygdaloid complex (AM), the external capsule (EC), and the zona incerta (ZI). The posterior border of the hypothalamus (panel F) is denoted by the appearance of the mammillary bodies (MB) and the posterior hypothalamic nucleus (PH). The mammillothalamic tract (MTT) is also shown.

medial border and into the cortex at the level of the rhinal fissure (see Fig. 4–11A). The small, irregular, and darkly staining clumps of cells observed throughout the amygdaloid complex are known as the **intercalated masses.** The thin line of cortical cells running ventrally and medially from the level of the rhinal fissure marks the boundary of the **pyriform cortex** (''pyriform'' means pear-shaped and refers to the shape of the outline of the cortex between the rhinal fissure and the base of the hypothalamus). The **lateral olfactory tract** is still seen as a compact bundle of fibers on the ventral surface of the brain, but at this level, it also spreads into a broad band of fibers running along the inferolateral surface of the pyriform cortex. The **olfactory tubercle** can still be seen medially to the lateral olfactory tract, although it is much more prominent in more anterior sections.

Immediately posterior to the level of the optic chiasm, the major nuclei of the amygdala are observable, although they are sometimes difficult to discern except through careful observation and comparison with more posterior sections. As shown in Figure 4–11(B), the corpus callosum is continuous with the **external capsule,** which marks the lateral border of the amygdaloid complex. The tear-shaped **lateral nucleus** of the amygdala lies just inside the internal capsule, with the more spherical **central nucleus** of the amygdala lying somewhat further medially. In most preparations, a small tuft of fibers, marking the beginning of the **stria terminalis,** can be seen at this level along with a small, crescent-shaped **intercalated mass.** The area between these structures and the hypothalamus is occupied by the **medial nucleus** of the amygdala, while the area immediately ventral to these structures is termed the **basal nucleus** of the amygdala (frequently divided into the **basolateral** and **basomedial** components, although the border between these is not clearly defined). Once again, the dark line of cells descending from the level of the rhinal fissure represents the **pyriform cortex.** The medial tip of this band of cells is associated with a larger clump of cells known as the **cortical nucleus** of the amygdala.

The nuclei that have been described are somewhat more obvious in the more posterior sections (see Fig. 4–11C). At this level, the optic tracts have turned dorsally and are seen as fiber masses projecting diagonally into the region between the base of the hypothalamus and the overlying cortex. The **medial nucleus** of the amygdala is situated on the lateral surface of the optic tract. The lateral nucleus is considerably larger and more clearly defined at this level, being separated from the medial nucleus by the spherically shaped central nucleus of the amygdala. The **cortical nucleus** is still present at the ventromedial border of the pyriform cortex. Nested among all of these structures are the **basal nuclei** of the amygdala, the medial and lateral divisions of which are still difficult to discern.

Still more posteriorly, the **stria terminalis** can be seen as it courses dorsally from the amygdala, and the entire amygdaloid complex becomes physically separated from the hypothalamus (see Fig. 4–11D). At this level, the **medial nucleus** forms the tip of the cortical lobe, the **cortical nucleus** is considerably larger, and the **lateral nucleus** is considerably smaller. Only the lateral division of the **basal nucleus** appears at this level. The area below the rhinal fissure which has been occupied by the amygdala and the pyriform cortex is shown as the **entorhinal cortex** at more posterior levels.

THE OLFACTORY SYSTEM

The structures of the olfactory system of the rat comprise a rather massive portion of the basal region of the forebrain. As shown in Figure 4–12, several of the major structures of this system are observable on the ventral surface of the brain. The most anterior portions of this system are the olfactory bulbs, which are frequently torn off unless special care is taken during removal of the brain from the skull. Two broad bands of fibers, the **lateral olfactory tracts,** can be seen coursing posteriorly from the olfactory bulbs along the ventral surface of the brain. These fibers project to the region of the amygdaloid complex, as will be seen later. The rather large islands which lie on either side of the optic nerves are the **olfactory tubercles.** The rather prominent fissure which forms the lateral border of these structures and runs posteriorly along the lateral edge of the pyriform cortex is the **rhinal sulcus.**

The series of sections show in Figure 4–13(A–D) show the cross-sectional configuration of these olfactory structures. In anterior sections, the olfactory bulbs have a laminated appearance. The band of fibers covering the lateral surface of the olfactory bulbs is the **lateral olfactory tract.** The bundle of fibers in the middle of the bulb is the **intermediate**

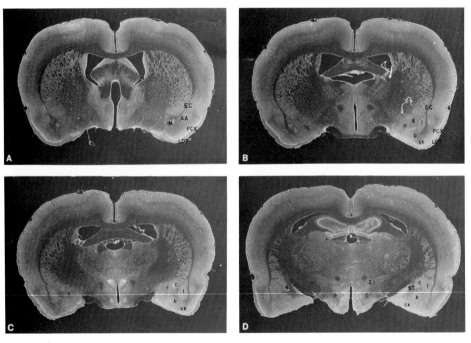

Fig. 4-11. Successively more posterior sections through the amygdaloid complex. The ill-defined anterior amygdaloid area (AA) and several intercalated masses (IM) are shown in panel A along with several adjacent structures, including the pyriform cortex (PCX), the lateral olfactory tract (LOT), and the olfactory tubercle. The major subdivisions of the amygdala (AM) are the lateral nucleus (1), the central nucleus (c), the basal nucleus (b), and the cortical nucleus (cx). Although these are identifiable in Panel B, they are much more clearly demarcated in more posterior regions (see panel C). Adjacent structures include the zona incerta (ZI) and the external capsule (EC). As shown in panel D, the fibers of the stria terminalis (ST) leave the posterior regions of the amygdaloid complex.

olfactory tract, which is surrounded by the **anterior olfactory nucleus.** The medial aspects of the bulbs are the so-called **granular layers** (see Fig. 4–13A).

In a more posterior plane, the medial olfactory tract is now termed the **anterior commissure,** with the **anterior olfactory nucleus** forming a more discrete structure located just medially to the fiber bundle. The **lateral olfactory tract** is more compact at this level, and the characteristic bumplike appearance of the **olfactory tubercle** is seen at the base of the brain. The dark line of cortical cells which begin at the level of the **rhinal sulcus** outline the **pyriform cortex** (see Fig. 4–13B).

Progressing more posteriorly, the anterior olfactory nucleus gives way to the very prominent **nucleus accumbens,** through which the **anterior commissure** passes somewhat eccentrically. The appearance of the olfactory tubercle, the lateral olfactory tract, and the pyriform cortex is similar to that of more anterior sections (see Fig. 4–13C).

At approximately the level of the optic chiasm, the fibers which originated in the intermediate olfactory tract cross via the **anterior commissure** and return to the olfactory bulbs via the contralateral intermediate olfactory tract. At this level, the **lateral olfactory tract** has once again flattened over the surface of the **pyriform cortex** and the **anterior amygdaloid area.** Some of the fibers of the **lateral olfactory tract** terminate on the cell bodies of the **nucleus of the lateral olfactory tract** (see Fig. 4–13D).

Unless one views serial coronal sections very carefully, it is easy to overlook another aspect of the anterior commissure—namely, that some of the fibers of this commissure

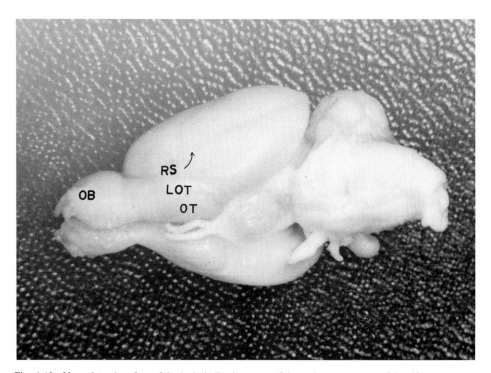

Fig. 4-12. Ventrolateral surface of the brain indicating some of the major components of the olfactory system. Included are the olfactory bulbs (OB), the lateral olfactory tracts (LOT), the olfactory tubercles (OT), and the rhinal sulcus (RS).

course laterally into cortical structures (the **intertemporal component**). This relationship (as well as the mutual connection between the olfactory bulbs) becomes much more obvious when viewed in the horizontal plane (see Fig. 4–14).

CORTICAL STRUCTURES

In addition to the subcortical structures that have been described, a rather substantial part of the cortex has also been included as a part of the limbic system. The most clearly demarcated region lies on the inferomedial aspect of the brain below the **rhinal sulcus** (see Fig. 4–15).

In the most anterior region, there is a smaller sulcus that descends from the rhinal sulcus to form a small triangular region of cortex known as the **prepyriform cortex.**

The terminology for the area posterior to the prepyriform cortex has not been entirely consistent. In some cases, the entire region beneath the rhinal sulcus is simply referred to as the **pyriform lobe.** More typically, this region is divided into an anterior portion called the pyriform cortex and a posterior portion called the **entorhinal cortex.** The division between these two regions corresponds to the border between the posterior amygdala and

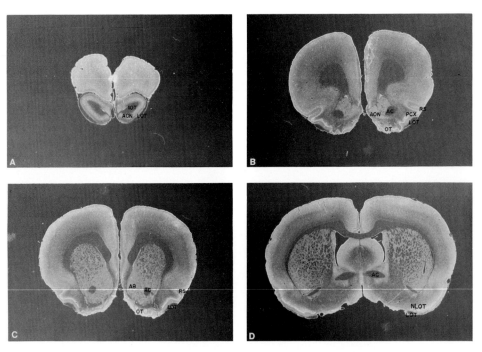

Fig. 4-13. Successively more posterior sections through the structures of the olfactory system. In anterior sections (panel A), the granular layers of the olfactory bulbs create a laminated appearance. The intermediate (IOT) and lateral (LOT) olfactory tracts are discrete bundles of fibers. The anterior olfactory nucleus (AON) surrounds the medial olfactory tract. More posteriorly (panel B), the intermediate olfactory tract is termed the "anterior commissure" (AC), and the olfactory tubercle (OT) is present along the ventral surface. Associated structures include the pyriform cortex (PCX) and the rhinal sulcus (RS). These structures continue more posteriorly (panels C and D) and are accompanied by the appearance of the nucleus accumbens (AB), the nucleus of the lateral olfactory tract (NLOT), and the anterior amygdaloid area.

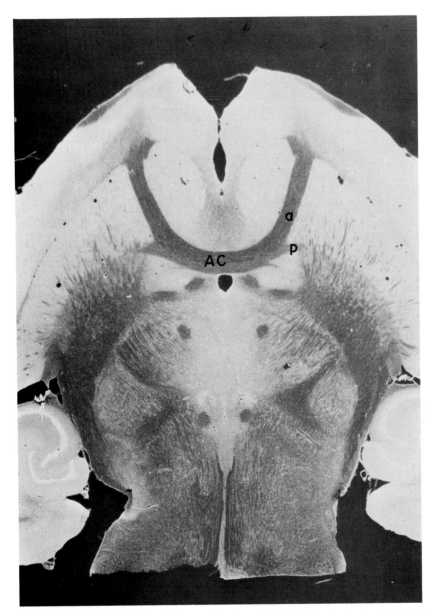

Fig. 4-14. Horizontal section through the ventral regions of the brain showing the two components of the anterior commissure (AC). The anterior portion (a) interconnects the olfactory bulbs, whereas the posterior branch (p) interconnects temporal cortical regions.

the ventral horn of the hippocampus. Additionally, some authors have used the term **periamygdaloid cortex** to refer to the region of the pyriform cortex that overlies the amygdala. Thus, for purposes of specificity, it would seem best to refer to successively more posterior regions of the area beneath the rhinal sulcus as follows: **prepyriform cortex, periamygdaloid cortex,** and **entorhinal cortex.**

A less clearly demarcated region is the **cingulate cortex,** which extends along the entire medial aspect of each hemisphere from the dorsal surface down to the corpus

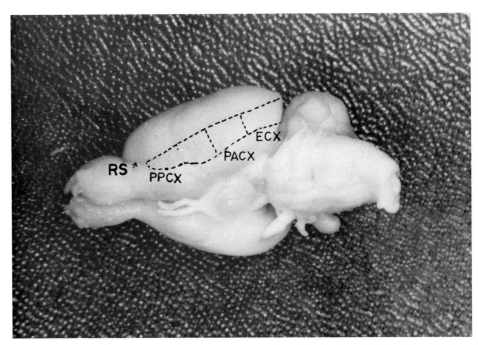

Fig. 4-15. The ventrolateral surface of the brain shows the large rhinal sulcus (RS) that forms the lateral boundary of the pyriform lobe. The approximate boundaries of the pyriform cortex (PCX), the periamygdaloid cortex (PACX), and the entorhinal cortex (ECS) are indicated.

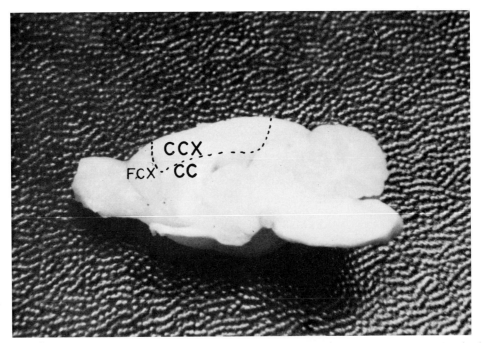

Fig. 4-16. The approximate outline of the cingulate cortex (CCX) is shown along the medial aspect of the cerebral hemisphere, just above the corpus callosum (CC). The most anterior regions are a part of the frontal cortex (FCX).

callosum. In other words, the cingulate gyri form the walls of the **longitudinal fissure.** The precise extent of the cingulate cortex, which can be determined only by detailed microscopic analysis, is approximately as indicated by the outline in Figure 4–16.

Another region that will later be included because of functional considerations is the **frontal cortex.** As indicated in Figure 4–17, the frontal cortex occupies the anterior and lateral aspects of the cortical mantle.

AREAS RELATED TO LIMBIC SYSTEM

The Thalamus

Although it is not usually considered as a part of the limbic system, certain parts of the thalamus interact with the traditional limbic system structures, a situation which necessitates a brief consideration of thalamic nuclei. The **thalamus** (which means inner chamber) is located deep in the center of the brain and is composed of a complex set of nuclei that have been divided and subdivided on the basis of both the detailed anatomical structure and the functions of the nuclei where known. For the present purposes, a rather simple description will suffice; the reader who is interested in greater detail should consult a more traditional anatomical text.

The easiest way to obtain a grasp of the general relationships of the major thalamic nuclei is to view a parasagittal section taken near the midline (about 0.5 mm laterally). As

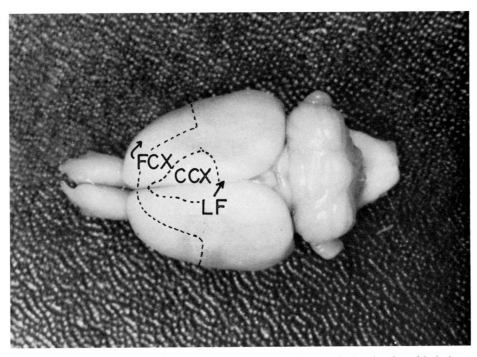

Fig. 4-17. The approximate outlines of the frontal cortex (FCX) are shown on the dorsal surface of the brain, on either side of the longitudinal fissure (LF). Additionally, a narrow strip of the cingulate cortex (CCX) can also be seen on the dorsal surface.

indicated in Figure 4–18, the thalamus is a large, nearly spherical mass in the center of the brain. Near the anterior border of the thalamus is a small round nucleus, the **anteromedial nucleus,** which receives fibers from the **mammillothalamic tract.** Although not clearly demarcated, the **parataenial nucleus** (named after its wormlike shape) curls up over the top of the anteromedial nucleus, and the **reuniens nucleus** angles down below the anteromedial nucleus. Most of the tissue behind the anteromedial nucleus represents the **medial** and **ventral** portions of the **medial thalamic nucleus.** The habenulo-interpeduncular tract (also called the fasciculus retroflexus) is surrounded by the **parafascicular nucleus.**

In coronal sections, the **medial thalamic nucleus** forms a half-circle beneath the stria medullaris bundles, with the **anteromedial nucleus** and fragments of the **mammillothalamic tract** being seen just beneath this half-circle. The **ventral thalamic nucleus** is sandwiched between the anteromedial nucleus and the large, curved **reticular nucleus,** which is adjacent to the internal capsule. The crescent-shaped **reuniens nucleus** lies on the midline just above the paraventricular nuclei of the hypothalamus. A small wedge of tissue located between the two stria medullaris bundles is known as the **paraventricular nucleus** of the thalamus (see Fig. 4–19A).

Moving more posteriorly behind the anteromedial nucleus, the large, semicircular **medial nucleus** becomes even more prominent and is bordered on either side by the **lateral nuclei.** The **ventral nuclei** are now quite large, leaving only thin bands of the reticular nuclei interposed between the ventral nuclei and the internal capsule. The **mammillothalamic tract** is seen as a pair of fiber bundles coursing through the lower portion of the thalamus (see Fig. 4–19B).

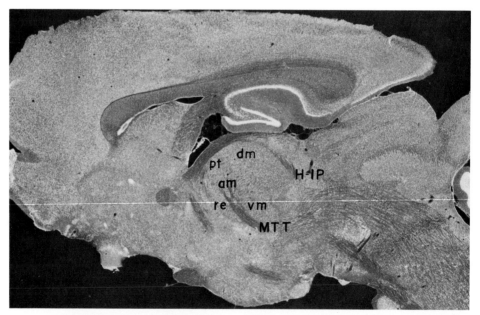

Fig. 4-18. Parasagittal view of the thalamus, near the midline, showing the anteromedial (am), dorsomedial (dm), and ventromedial (vm) nuclei of the thalamus. The major fiber tracts are the habenulo-interpeduncular tract (H-IP) and the mammillothalamic tract (MTT). Smaller nuclei include the parataenial nucleus (pt) and the reuniens nucleus (re).

The Tegmentum

The term **tegmentum** means covering and refers to the fact that this region of the brain overlies the cerebral peduncles. The major regions that are of interest with respect to limbic system connections can be seen in coronal section at the level of the **interpeduncular nucleus.** Prominent landmarks at this level are the broad bands of fibers at the base of the brain known as the **cerebral peduncles,** the large darkly staining region known as the **substantia nigra** (dark substance) which lies just above the peduncles, and the diagonally oriented fiber bundles of the **medial lemniscus** (see Fig. 4–20A). The smaller bundles of fibers located on either side of the interpeduncular nucleus are the **mammillary peduncles.** The large, fan-shaped region surrounding the **cerebral aqueduct** (of Sylvius) is referred to as the central gray. The two small tufts of fibers near the midline at the base of the central gray substance are the **medial longitudinal fasciculi.** The fibers that crisscross the midline between the central gray and the interpeduncular nucleus represent the **dorsal** and **ventral tegmental decussations.** The large areas on either side of the central gray represent the **reticular formation.**

In more posterior sections, the fibers of the **pons** are seen coursing across the base of the brain, the dark areas just above the fibers near the midline being the **pontine nuclei** (see Fig. 4–20B). The band of fibers extending vertically on the midline is called the

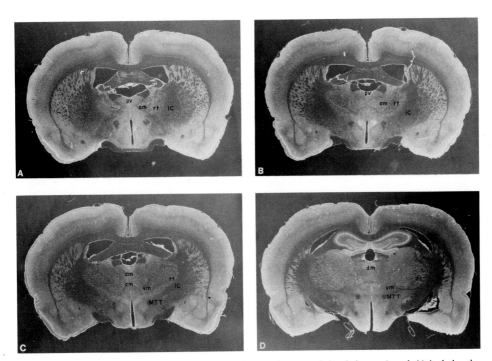

Fig. 4-19. Coronal sections through the thalamus. The anterior part of the thalamus (panel A) includes the anteromedial nucleus (am). The internal capsule (IC) forms the border of the thalamus. Within this border, the ventromedial nucleus (vm), the reticular nucleus (rt), and the periventricular nucleus (pv) of the thalamus may also be seen. More posteriorly, some of these same structures may be seen, with the dorsomedial (dm) and ventromedial (vm) nuclei being especially large. The mammillothalamic tract can be seen in cross section along the ventral aspect of the thalamus.

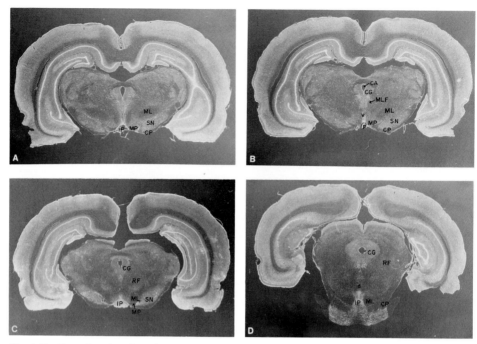

Fig. 4-20. Coronal sections through the tegmentum, denoted by the presence of the cerebral peduncles (CP), the mammillary peduncles (MP), and substantia nigra (SN), and the interpeduncular nucleus (IP), which is partially missing. Additional landmarks include the medial lemniscus (ML), the cerebral aqueduct (CA), the medial longitudinal fasciculus (MLF), the dorsal (d) and ventral (v) tegmental decussations, the reticular formation (RF), and the central gray (CG), which surrounds the cerebral aqueduct.

raphe (which means seam); this represents a concentration of fibers crossing the midline. Immediately above the raphe, on the midline, is the **medial raphe nucleus,** which is bordered on either side by the reticular formation. The darkly stained nucleus within the lower portion of the central gray region is the **dorsal raphe nucleus.** At this level, the **medial longitudinal fasciculi** form more distinct bundles at the base of the central gray.

The Fornix System and Related Hippocampal Connections

5

INTRODUCTION

One of the most prominent fiber systems of the forebrain is the fornix, which becomes obvious at the level of the anterior poles of the hippocampus. At this level, the total fornix bundle is actually composed of the fibers of the fimbria and the more medially located fibers of the dorsal fornix. From this point of convergence, the fibers arch downward (''fornix'' means arch) and split into two components: a rather diffuse component that descends through the septum anterior to the level of the anterior commissure into the preoptic area and a more compact postcommissural component that descends to the mammillary bodies. The series of coronal and parasagittal sections in Figure 5–1 shows the general topography of this fiber bundle.

The fornix is a bundle of fibers which forms partially reciprocating connections between the hippocampus, septum, hypothalamus, thalamus, and midbrain. As such, it represents one of the major fiber systems involved with the interconnection of limbic system structures. Because of the complexity of this system, there are numerous ways in which the description of the fiber projections can be organized. One way would be to consider separately the pre- and postcommissural components of the system. Another method would be to consider the system in terms of the separate origins of the fibers which make up the system. Or the projection pathway of the fibers could be used as the criterion. For the present purposes, the description will be based upon the projection pathway of the fibers and will be divided into three sections: (1) the dorsal fornix system, (2) the fimbrial system, and (3) other hippocampal connections. The reader may gain additional insight into the organization of this system by reorganizing the connections described in terms of the other types of divisions that have been noted. Much of the following detailed description of these systems is based upon the technical publications of Guillery (1956), Lorente de Nó (1934), Nauta (1956, 1958), Nauta and Haymaker (1969), Raisman (1966), Raisman, Cowan, & Powell (1965, 1966), Hjorth-Simonsen (1971, 1973), and Gottlieb and Cowan (1973).

53

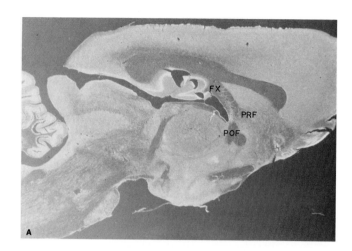

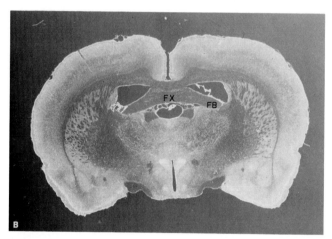

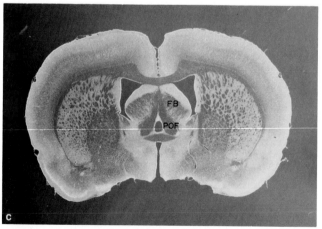

Fig. 5-1. The parasagittal section in panel A shows the main body of the fornix (FX) splitting into the diffuse precommissural component (PRF) and the compact postcommissural columns (POF) of the fornix. The coronal section through the main body of the fornix (panel B) also shows the more laterally located fimbria (FB). More anterior sections (panel C) show the descending columns of the postcommissural fornix.

The connections of the hippocampus are greatly complicated by its spatial organization. Unlike other structures which tend to be organized into fairly discrete nuclei that are situated side by side, the hippocampus is a complex, layered structure that appears to have been rolled into a tube like a jelly roll. Anatomists have attempted to divide this complex structure into units on the basis of the detailed structure and organization of the cells. This cytoarchitectonic approach (cf. Lorente de Nó, 1934) has resulted in four major subdivisions of the hippocampus being categorized (cornu Ammonis [CA]). Examples of the defining criteria follow:

CA 1: Pyramidal cells give rise to side branches in stratum radiatum.
CA 2: Receive collaterals from the presubiculum.
CA 3: Give rise to Schaffer collaterals.
CA 4: Give rise to Schaffer collaterals but have no basket complexes.

This type of detailed microscopic analysis of cellular connections goes well beyond the scope of this text, so the approximate locations of these cell populations will be outlined. Figure 5–2 shows several drawings of the hippocampal complex with the approxi-

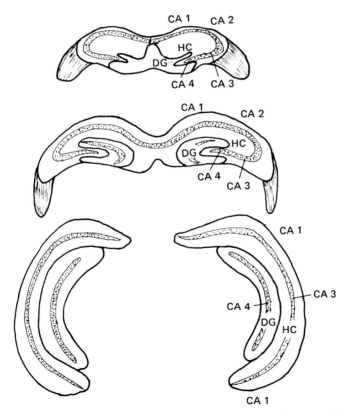

Fig. 5-2. Highly schematized representation of the approximate location of the various cytoarchitectonic fields (CA 1 through CA 4) of the hippocampal complex (HC) and dentate gyrus (DG).

mate locations of these cellular fields. The spatial organization is obviously complex, but certain useful generalities can be made: **Areas CA 1** and **CA 2** are largely represented in the dorsal regions of the hippocampus, with area CA 2 being closely associated with the fibers of the fimbria. By contrast, the bulk of **areas CA 3** and **CA 4** are located within the large descending horns of the ventral hippocampus. These generalities hardly do justice to the exquisite drawings and descriptions of Lorente de No' and more recent investigators but will serve as anchor points for the descriptions of pathways that follow.

THE DORSAL FORNIX SYSTEM

The dorsal fornix represents the medial aspect of the entire fornix bundle at the level of the anterior thalamus. The fibers which make up the dorsal fornix arise almost entirely from the pyramidal cells of the anterior portion of **layer CA 1,** although there is also a smaller component of fibers arising from cells in the posterior portion of CA 1.

The fibers originating from cells in the anterior portion of CA 1 course through the dorsal fornix and then descend exclusively in the **postcommissural** columns of the fornix. Some of these fibers leave the columns of the fornix and turn posteriorly to terminate in the **anterior thalamic nucleus,** while other fibers continue ventrally to terminate primarily in the posterior parts of the **medial** and **lateral mammillary nuclei.** Additionally, there may be a smaller component of fibers which turns dorsally and posteriorly from a point just above the mammillary bodies to terminate in the **midbrain.** There is little or no evidence for the termination within the septal nuclei of any of these fibers arising from CA 1.

The second and smaller component of the dorsal fornix arises from the pyramidal

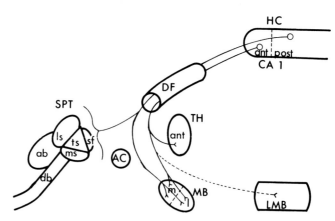

Fig. 5-3. Summary of the projections of the dorsal fornix. HC = hippocampus (ant = anterior and post = posterior regions of area CA 1), DF = dorsal fornix, SPT = septum (ls = lateral septum, ts = triangular nucleus, sf = septofimbrial nucleus, ms = medial nucleus, ab = accumbens nucleus, db = diagonal band), AC = anterior commissure, TH = thalamus (anterior portions), MB = mammillary body (m = medial, l = lateral), LMB = limbic midbrain.

cells of the **posterior** part of CA 1. (Some of these fibers also pass through the fimbria, but there is no evidence for differential distribution.) These fibers show a considerably more diversified distribution than do the fibers from the anterior portion of CA 1. Some of these fibers terminate in the anterior portions of the **medial** and **lateral mammillary nuclei** but apparently do not project to either the midbrain or the anterior thalamus. Unlike the fibers from the anterior portion of CA 1, the fibers arising from the more posterior regions show a rather extensive precommissural projection to virtually all parts of the septal complex; specifically, these fibers terminate in the **septofimbrial nucleus,** the **medial septal nucleus,** the **diagonal band,** the **accumbens nucleus,** and the ventromedial aspect of the **lateral septal nucleus.**

A summary of these projections is shown in Figure 5–3.

THE FIMBRIAL SYSTEM

The term "fimbria" means fringe and is descriptive of the fact that the fimbria is comprised of a bundle of fibers which follows the ventrolateral border of the hippocampus for some distance before coming into juxtaposition with the fibers of the dorsal fornix. As indicated in the previous section, there is a small group of fibers from the posterior portion of CA 1 that projects through the fimbria, but the vast majority of these fibers arise from the pyramidal cells of CA 2 and of CA 3 and 4.

The fibers arising from **area CA 2** show a very limited distribution, traveling in the **postcommissural columns** of the fornix and terminating exclusively in the **anterior thalamic nucleus** and the **medial mammillary nucleus.**

The fibers arising from **areas CA 3 and CA 4** (differential distribution of the two divisions has not been established) also show a somewhat limited distribution, being entirely within the **precommissural fornix.** These precommissural fibers project to the dorsolateral aspect of the **lateral septal nucleus,** the nucleus of the **diagonal band,** the **arcuate nucleus,** and via the medial forebrain bundle to the **preoptic nucleus.** The fibers that pass through the septum to terminate in the preoptic area are joined by fibers arising in the septum, some of which bypass the preoptic region to project caudally into the midbrain. Apparently none of these midbrain projections is of hippocampal origin. The bundle of hippocampal and septal fibers that descends into the preoptic area is sometimes termed the **medial corticohypothalamic tract.**

The **subiculum** also gives rise to a few fibers which project via the fimbria to the **supraoptic** nucleus of the hypothalamus. The dentate gyrus apparently does not give rise to an extrahippocampal projection.

In addition to the efferent projections of the hippocampus, the fimbria also contains a substantial number of fibers that arise from the **medial septal nucleus** and the nucleus of the **diagonal band** and terminate in **areas CA 3 and CA 4,** as well as in the **dentate gyrus.**

A summary of this system is shown in Figure 5–4.

It should be noted that some recent results of other anatomists (Siegel, Edinger, & Ogami, 1974) have indicated that the projections of the hippocampus are not related to the cytoarchitectonic subdivisions. Instead, it may be organized in a relatively simpler topographical fashion, the dorsal hippocampus projecting to the medial septal nucleus and the ventral hippocampus projecting to the lateral septal nuclei. The interested reader should check up-to-date primary sources for the current status of this argument.

OTHER HIPPOCAMPAL CONNECTIONS

Connections with Entorhinal Cortex

As mentioned, the hippocampus receives direct inputs from only two sources: fibers arising in the medial septal nucleus and the nucleus of the diagonal band that converge on the hippocampus via the fimbria and also from the entorhinal cortex.

The **entorhinal cortex** contributes fibers to the hippocampus via two components: The **direct temporo-ammonic tract** sends fibers arising from the lateral aspects of entorhinal area through the subiculum to terminate primarily in **areas CA 1** and **CA 2** but with some terminations in **CA 3** and the **dentate gyrus** as well. The **temporo-alvear tract** arises from cells in the medial aspects of the entorhinal cortex and courses medially and dorsally to enter the alveus, from which it terminates only in **CA 1** of the hippocampus and in the pyramidal cells of the subiculum.

In addition to the contributions of the entorhinal cortex to the hippocampus, there is also a projection of fibers to the **contralateral subiculum** via the crossed **temporo-ammonic tract,** which decussates in the **dorsal hippocampal commissure** (dorsal psalterium). Finally, it should be noted that recent observations have revealed that **area CA 3** gives rise to fibers that project systematically (though not entirely topographically) to the entorhinal cortex (cf. Hjorth-Simonsen, 1971).

A summary of these projections is shown in Figure 5–5.

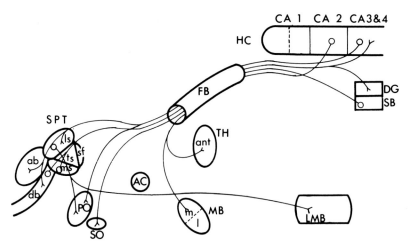

Fig. 5-4. Summary of the projections of the fimbria. HC = hippocampus, DG = dentate gyrus, SB = subiculum, FB = fimbria, SPT = septum (ls = lateral septum, ts = triangular nucleus, sf = septofimbrial nucleus, ab = accumbens nucleus, ms = medial septum, db = diagonal band), PO = preoptic region, SO = supraoptic nucleus, AC = anterior commissure, TH = thalamus (ant = anterior nucleus), MB = mammillary body (l = lateral, m = medial), LMB = limbic midbrain.

Most of the interconnections among the various regions of the hippocampus are probably via short-axon relays which pass through the closely layered structures of the hippocampus. Such connections, although undoubtedly important, are difficult to describe and cannot be studied by the current procedures for degeneration staining. Such connections must be established by the tedious method of studying normal material stained, for example, by the Golgi technique. There are, however, four long-fiber systems which are known to interconnect hippocampal structures:

1. *Collaterals from CA 3 and CA 4.* The axon collaterals from **areas CA 3** and **CA 4,** known as Schaffer collaterals, project to **areas CA 1** and **CA 2.**

2. *Collaterals from CA 1 and CA 2.* Axon collaterals from **areas CA 1** and **CA 2** project primarily to the **subiculum** and apparently do not contribute a reciprocating connection to areas CA 3 and CA 4.

3. *Dentate–hippocampal projection.* The granule cells of the **dentate gyrus** give rise to many fibers which terminate in **areas CA 3** and **CA 4.**

4. *Hippocampal–dentate projection.* There may also be a reciprocating projection from the hippocampus to the dentate gyrus, but the precise origin and course of this projection has not been determined.

A summary of these projections is shown in Figure 5–6.

Hippocampal Commissures

There are two commissural systems that interconnect the two hippocampi:

1. The **ventral hippocampal commissure** (ventral psalterium) can be seen in gross dissection as a broad band of fibers stretching across the underside of the two horns of the hippocampal formation. It contains the fibers of the fimbria, which distribute to the contralateral fimbria and then project to virtually all levels of the hippocampal formation.

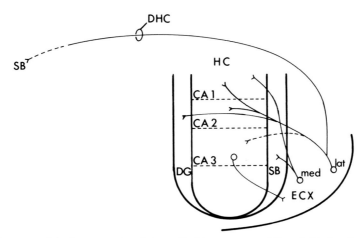

Fig. 5-5. Summary of the interconnections between the hippocampus and the entorhinal cortex. ECX = entorhinal cortex (med = medial, lat = lateral), SB = subiculum, DG = dentate gyrus, HC = hippocampus, DHC = dorsal hippocampal commissure.

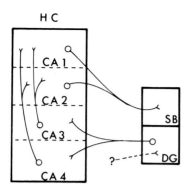

Fig. 5-6. Summary of the association connections within the hippocampus. HC = hippocampus, SB = subiculum, DG = dentate gyrus.

2. The **dorsal hippocampal commissure** (dorsal psalterium) is a continuation of fibers from the alveus, which forms a compact flat band of fibers that cross just beneath the corpus callosum. Although there is some degree of specificity, the two commissures are interconnected so that most regions that give rise to crossed projections reach the contralateral side via both commissural systems (cf. Blackstad, 1956).

These two commissures can be seen in Figure 5–7 and Figure 5–8.

The interconnections that are made via the two commissures are somewhat complex and, for the most part, are not strictly homotopic. Although **area CA 3** of the hippocampus forms a symmetrical and homotopic connection with the same subfields on the contralateral side, the remaining fibers do not appear to be commissural in the strict sense of the term. In addition to the homotopic projections from **area CA 3** of the hippocampus, these cells also give rise to fibers that terminate in **area CA 1** of the opposite side. Fibers that arise from the **CA 3** pyramidal cells of the **dentate gyrus** project to the granule cells of the contralateral dentate gyrus. With respect to these crossed projections, Gottlieb and Cowan (1973) have pointed out an important feature of the organization of these systems: In all cases that they have studied, cells that give rise to crossed projections also project to

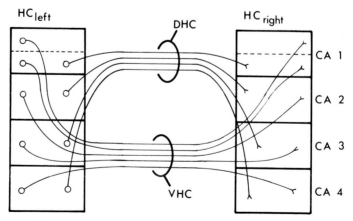

Fig. 5-7. Summary of the hippocampal commissures. HC = hippocampus, DHC = dorsal hippocampal commissure, VHC = ventral hippocampal commissure.

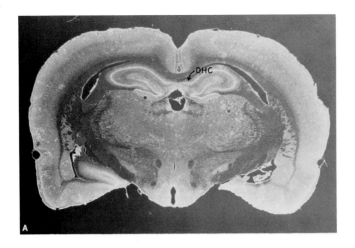

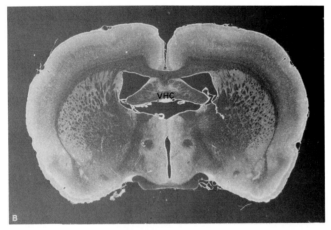

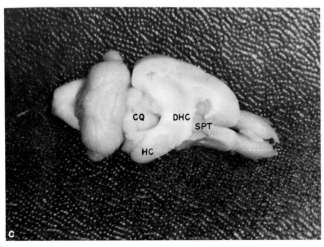

Fig. 5-8. Panels A and B show coronal views of the dorsal (DHC) and ventral (VHC) commissures of the hippocampus. Panel C shows a dorsal view of the dissected hippocampal complex, indicating the broad band of fibers that form the dorsal hippocampal commissure. The hippocampus (HC), septum (SPT), and corpora quadrigemina (CQ) serve as additional points of reference.

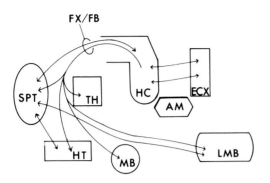

Fig. 5-9. General overview of the relationship of the hippocampus to other regions of the brain. HC = hippocampus, FX = fornix, SPT = septum, HT = hypothalamus, AM = amygdala, ECX = entorhinal cortex, LMB = limbic midbrain, MB = mammillary bodies.

the homotopic region of the same side. Thus, even in the case of crossed projections, there remains a high degree of symmetry in the regions of termination.

A summary of these projections is shown in Figure 5–7.

SUMMARY

The fornix system represents the major pathway for the interconnection of the septohippocampal complex with the hypothalamus and midbrain (see Fig. 5–9). The septum and hippocampus share internal circuitry that suggests a high degree of interaction. The bi-directional connections between these forebrain structures and the sensory, visceral, and motor aspects of the hypothalamus and midbrain may provide a clue to the possible function of this system.

Connections of the Stria Medullaris and Habenulae

6

INTRODUCTION

The stria medullaris is a fiber system which becomes evident just posterior to the septal region, from which point it arches dorsally and caudally along either side of the midline to the habenular nuclei. This fiber bundle interconnects a variety of structures from the septal, hypothalamic, and olfactory regions with more posteriorly located nuclei of the thalamus and the tegmentum.

The details of these connections will now be described. The reader who is interested in additional and more detailed coverage of this material should refer to Cragg (1961), Marburg (1944), or Nauta and Haymaker (1969).

THE SEPTAL CONTRIBUTION

Because of the obvious physical relationship of the septum, stria medullaris, and habenular nuclei, the stria medullaris is often considered to be principally a septohabenular system. Although the septal nuclei in fact contribute to the stria medullaris, the distribution to the habenular nuclei is somewhat restricted and other sources also provide massive input into this system.

Virtually all of the cell bodies of the septal nuclei that give rise to fibers passing through the stria medullaris are located in the posterior one-third of the septum, i.e., from the triangular nucleus and the posterior portions of the medial and lateral septal nuclei. The fibers arising from these nuclei ascend with the fornix fibers and then turn posteriorly through the dorsal portion of the stria medullaris bundle, and most of them terminate in the **medial habenular nucleus** of the ipsilateral side. Approximately 20% of the fibers which terminate in the medial habenula cross over to the contralateral side via the **habenular commissure.** (As indicated in Figure 6–1, another massive fiber system, the fornix, is

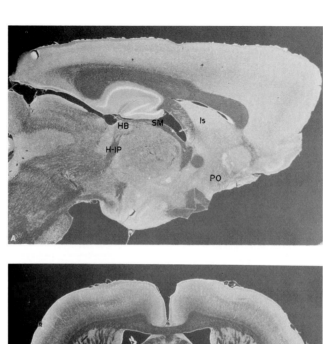

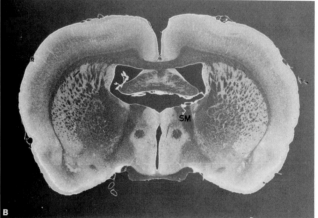

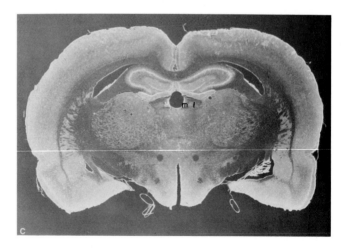

Fig. 6-1. The parasagittal view (panel A) of the stria medullaris (SM) shows the major structures associated with this system. Included are the lateral septum (ls), preoptic area (PO), lateral habenula (HB), and habenulo-interpeduncular tract (H-IP) as it descends toward the interpeduncular nucleus. Panels B and C show coronal sections of the stria medullaris (SM) as it collects fibers near the posterior border of the septum, before projecting posteriorly to the medial (m) and lateral (l) divisions of the habenula.

passing through the posterior septum near the points of origin of the stria medullaris fibers. However, the fornix apparently does not contribute fibers to the stria medullaris.)

In addition to this major projection from the posterior septum to the medial habenula, a few of these fibers leave the main stria medullaris bundle and course ventrally through the medial habenular nucleus to terminate in the **paraventricular nucleus** of the **thalamus.** A second group of fibers descends via the **habenulo-interpeduncular tract** either to terminate in the **interpeduncular nucleus** or to split into a third group of fibers that courses posteriorly to various levels of the **reticular formation.**

A summary of these projections is shown in Figure 6–2.

THE PREOPTIC CONTRIBUTION

The preoptic area of the hypothalamus contributes a large and somewhat complicated component of fibers to the stria medullaris. Cell bodies in the **olfactory tubercle** and anterior **preoptic region** (and perhaps from the **medial forebrain bundle,** see Fig. 6–3) course upward, passing just beneath the anterior commissure, and enter the dorsal region of the stria medullaris at the level of the fornix columns, i.e., these fibers intermingle with the fibers of septal origin that have been described. From this point, most of the fibers continue posteriorly to terminate in the **lateral habenular nucleus** of the ipsilateral side, although there are a few fibers that leave the stria medullaris before reaching the habenula to course ventrally into the **dorsomedial nucleus** of the **thalamus.** Apparently, none of these fibers enters the medial habenula. This fiber system projecting to the lateral habenula is particularly obvious in rodents and has been termed the **lateral olfac-tohabenular tract** (e.g., Nauta & Haymaker, 1969).

Those fibers which do not terminate directly in the lateral habenula either cross over to the contralateral side or course ventrally into the **habenulo-interpeduncular tract.**

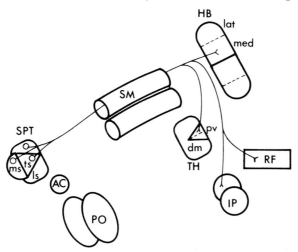

Fig. 6-2. Summary of the septal contribution to the stria medullaris. SPT = septum (ms = medial septum, ls = lateral septum, ts = triangular nucleus), SM = stria medullaris, HB = habenula (lat = lateral nucleus, med = medial nucleus), pv = paraventricular nucleus of the thalamus (TH), dm = dorsomedial nucleus of the thalamus, RF = reticular formation, IP = interpeduncular nucleus, AC = anterior commissure, PO = preoptic region.

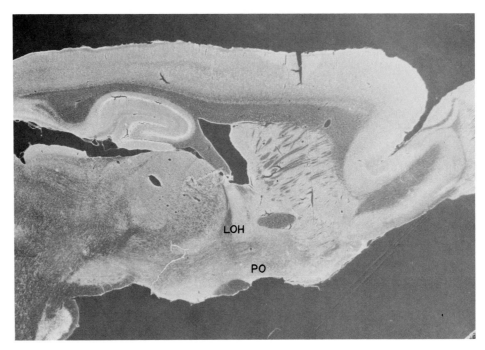

Fig. 6-3. Parasagittal view showing the convergence of fibers from the preoptic region (PO) and from more laterally located regions of the cortex. This bundle of fibers, which contributes to the formation of the stria medullaris, is sometimes referred to as the lateral olfactohabenular tract (LOH) in rodents.

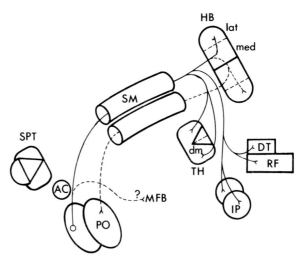

Fig. 6-4. Summary of the preoptic contribution to the stria medullaris. PO = preoptic region, MFB = medial forebrain bundle, SM = stria medullaris, HB = habenula (lat = lateral nucleus, med = medial nucleus), dm = dorsomedial nucleus of the thalamus (TH), IP = interpeduncular nucleus, DT = dorsal tegmentum, RF = reticular formation.

These descending fibers are divided into three components: (1) Some of the fibers leave the habenulo-interpeduncular tract to enter the posterior portion of the **dorsomedial nucleus** of the **thalamus.** (2) Other fibers continue ventrally to a point just above the **interpeduncular nuclei,** form a partial decussation, and apparently terminate both ipsilaterally and contralaterally in these nuclei. (3) The remaining fibers leave the habenulo-interpeduncular tract at the point of the decussation and project diffusely in a posterior direction to terminate in the **reticular formation** and the **dorsal tegmentum.**

The fibers from the preoptic area that enter the **habenular commissure** can be divided into two components. Some of these fibers simply terminate in the **lateral habenula** of the **contralateral** side. The remaining fibers course **anteriorly** through the contralateral stria medullaris and then ventrally beneath the anterior commissure to terminate in the **preoptic area** and the **substantia innominata.** Thus, there is a recurrent loop of the preoptic projection system which returns to the **contralateral preoptic area.**

A summary of the preoptic projection system is shown in Figure 6–4.

THE THALAMIC CONTRIBUTION

As indicated, most of the fibers of the stria medullaris arise from the preoptic region and the posterior regions of the septum. As this bundle of fibers courses posteriorly along the dorsal aspect of the thalamus, it receives additional fibers from the thalamic nuclei. Specifically, the **anteroventral** and **reticular nuclei** of the **thalamus** (see Fig. 6–5) give rise to fibers that enter the dorsal region of the stria medullaris and eventually terminate in

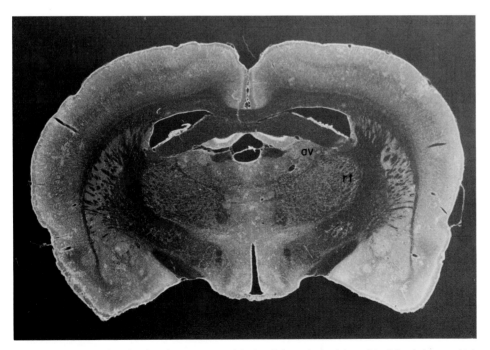

Fig. 6-5. Coronal section showing the anteroventral (av) and the reticular (rt) nuclei of the thalamus which contribute to the stria medullaris.

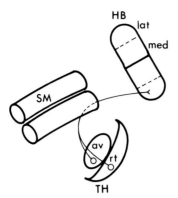

Fig. 6-6. Summary of the thalamic projections through the stria medullaris. av = anteroventral nucleus of the thalamus (TH), rt = reticular thalamic nucleus, SM = stria medullaris, HB = habenula (lat = lateral, med = medial).

the **lateral habenular nucleus** of the ipsilateral side. There are apparently no projections to the medial habenula, the habenulo-interpeduncular tract, or to contralateral structures. (It should be noted that although some of these fibers are in close juxtaposition to the mammillothalamic tract at the point of their origin, this hypothalamic fiber system does not project to either the stria medullaris or the habenula.)

A summary of this projection is shown in Figure 6–6.

THE AMYGDALOID CONTRIBUTION

Although the amygdala does not contribute heavily to the stria medullaris–habenula system, a few fibers have been found to leave the **stria terminalis** and enter the lateral portion of the stria medullaris at the level of the anterior thalamus. The fibers project posteriorly, where some of the fibers terminate in the **lateral habenula,** while others project to the medial portion of the **dorsomedial nucleus** of the thalamus. A few of the fibers cross to the contralateral side via the **habenular commissure** to terminate in the

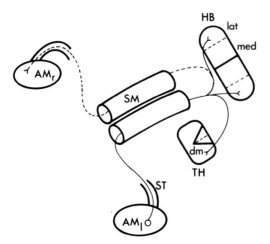

Fig. 6-7. Summary of the amygdaloid projections through the stria medullaris. AM = amygdala (l = left, r = right), SM = stria medullaris, HB = habenula (lat = lateral, med = medial), dm = dorsomedial nucleus of the thalamus (TH).

lateral habenula and (perhaps) project anteriorly in the stria medullaris to rejoin the **contralateral stria terminalis.**

A summary of this projection is shown in Figure 6–7.

THE CONTRIBUTION OF THE INTERPEDUNCULAR NUCLEUS

In the projection systems that have been described, it has been noted that several systems involve fibers which descend via the habenulo-interpeduncular tract into various midbrain areas, most notably the interpeduncular nucleus. This tract, like most others, is a reciprocating pathway and contains a large number of fibers which appear to have their origins in the **interpeduncular nucleus.** These fibers ascend in the **habenulo-interpeduncular tract** and project mainly into the region of the **lateral habenular nucleus** (but not the medial), although a few fibers leave this tract to enter the posterior portion of the **dorsomedial nucleus** of the thalamus. Of the fibers which project to the region of the habenula, some of these terminate in the **lateral habenular nucleus** while others project anteriorly via the dorsal aspect of the **stria medullaris** to terminate in the **preoptic area** and the **substantia innominata.**

A summary of these projections is shown in Figure 6–8.

PROJECTIONS FROM THE MEDIAL HABENULA

A heavy projection of fibers which originates in or passes through the medial habenula courses posteroventrally via the ipsilateral **habenulo-interpeduncular tract** to a point just above the interpeduncular nucleus, at which point a partial decussation occurs (see Fig. 6–9). These fibers then terminate mainly in the **interpeduncular nucleus,** although some of the fibers project posteriorly into the **central gray** area at the level of the dorsal tegmental nucleus.

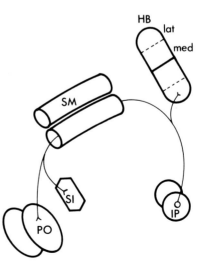

Fig. 6-8. Summary of the contribution of the interpeduncular nucleus to the stria medullaris. IP = interpeduncular nucleus, HB = habenula (med = medial, lat = lateral), SM = stria medullaris, SI = substantia innominata, PO = preoptic region.

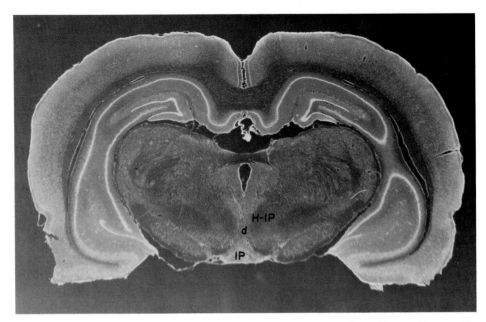

Fig. 6-9. The habenulo-interpeduncular tract descends to the interpeduncular nucleus, with some fibers crossing just above the nucleus to form a decussation. IP = interpeduncular nucleus, H-IP = habenulo-interpeduncular tract, d = decussation.

Fibers arising from the medial habenular nucleus apparently do not project anteriorly into the stria medullaris, nor do they project to the contralateral habenular nuclei via the habenular commissure.

A summary of this projection is shown in Figure 6–10.

PROJECTIONS FROM THE LATERAL HABENULA

The fibers which originate in or pass through the lateral habenula show a different and somewhat more complicated pattern of projection than those of the medial habenula.

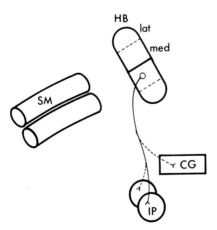

Fig. 6-10. Summary of the projections from the medial habenula. HB = habenula (med = medial nucleus, lat = lateral nucleus), CG = central gray, IP = interpeduncular nucleus.

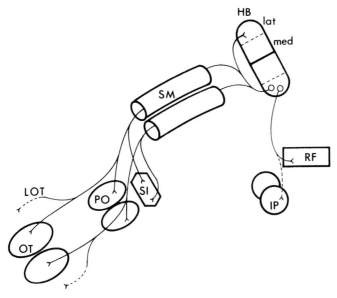

Fig. 6-11. Summary of the projections from the lateral habenula. HB = habenula (lat = lateral nucleus, med = medial nucleus), RF = reticular formation, IP = interpeduncular nucleus, SM = stria medullaris, SI = substantia innominata, PO = preoptic area, LOT = lateral olfactory tract, OT = olfactory tubercle.

The descending projection into the **habenulo-interpeduncular tract** is less prominent than that of the medial habenula, and after partial decussation most of these fibers project dorsally and posteriorly to terminate at various levels of the **reticular formation.** Apparently, only a few of these fibers enter the interpeduncular nucleus.

A further contrast to the medial system is that there is a heavy projection of fibers to

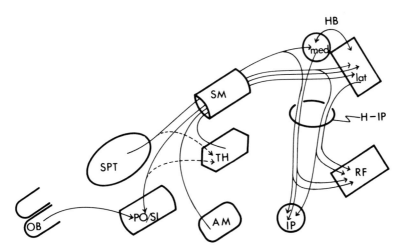

Fig. 6-12. An overview of the stria medullaris–habenula system. OB = olfactory bulbs, SPT = septum, PO/SI = preoptic/substantia innominata region, SM = stria medullaris, TH = thalamus, AM = amygdala, HB = habenula (med = medial, lat = lateral), H-IP = habenulo-interpeduncular tract, IP = interpeduncular nucleus, RF = reticular formation.

the **contralateral lateral habenula.** Following this crossed projection, there are many fibers which enter the **stria medullaris** and course anteriorly to terminate bilaterally in the **preoptic area** and the **substantia innominata.** Additionally, some of these fibers proceed even further anteriorly to terminate in the **olfactory tubercle** and the **nucleus of the lateral olfactory tract.**

A summary of this projection is shown in Figure 6–11.

SUMMARY

In summary, the stria medullaris–habenula system provides a rather massive system of fibers which interconnects structures along virtually the entire longitudinal extent of the brain. As summarized in Figure 6–12, the medial and lateral portions of this system appear to be relatively independent. The medial system involves connections between the posterior septal region and the medial habenular nucleus. The lateral system involves connections between the olfactory–preoptic areas and the lateral habenula. Both parts of this system project to the interpeduncular nucleus and to the midbrain. Two additional peculiarities are that only the lateral habenulae appear to be interconnected via the habenular commissure, and only the lateral nuclei receive a reciprocating connection from the interpeduncular nucleus.

The Stria Terminalis, The Ventral Amygdaloid Pathways, and Related Amygdaloid Connections

7

INTRODUCTION

The amygdala is composed of a group of nuclei located just beneath the cortical mantle of the inferior temporal lobe. This region is interconnected with cortical regions, the olfactory system, and portions of the thalamus and hypothalamus.

The most obvious fiber system associated with the amygdaloid area is the stria terminalis. This band of fibers leaves the dorsal region of the amygdala, arches up and over the thalamus, and then descends to terminate in several nuclei of the thalamus and hypothalamus. This rather circuitous and indirect pathway is two or three times longer than would be required by a direct route to the same regions of termination.

In addition to this rather indirect route, there is a more direct ventral projection from the amygdala which terminates in some of the same areas as the stria terminalis, as well as some thalamic structures. This pathway may be as large as the stria terminalis but, being diffuse, is difficult to trace.

Finally, it should be pointed out that the amygdala receives a fair number of fibers from the olfactory system, these connections providing some of the initial reasons for the term "rhinencephalon."

Much of the description of these projections which will be presented below is based upon more detailed articles by Cowan, Raisman, and Powell (1965), de Olmos (1972), Hall (1972), Heimer and Nauta (1969), and Nauta and Haymaker (1969). The histological sections shown in Figure 7–1 give an overview of the pathway followed by the stria terminalis.

73

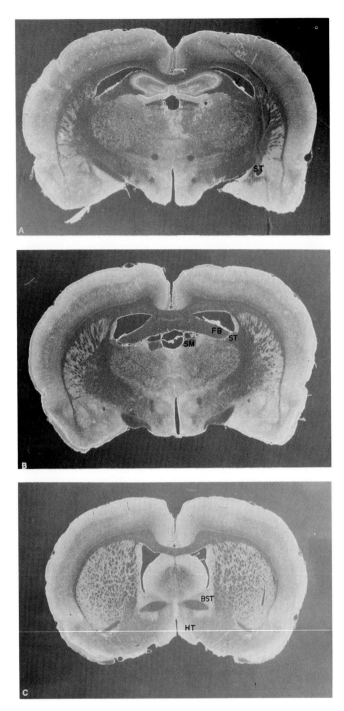

Fig. 7-1. Successively more anterior sections showing the route of the stria terminalis (ST). The fibers of the stria terminalis are collected in the posterior regions of the amygdala (panel A) and travel upwards to the base of the third ventricle (V). From this point, the bundle of fibers turns anteriorly and courses alongside the stria medullaris (SM) and fimbria (FB), as shown in panel B. The fibers then descend in the region between the septum and the thalamus, forming the bed nucleus of the stria terminalis (BST) before terminating (panel C) in various regions of the hypothalamus (HT).

DORSAL COMPONENT OF STRIA TERMINALIS

75

STRIA TERMINALIS,
VENTRAL
AMYGDALOID
PATHWAYS,
AND AMYGDALOID
CONNECTIONS

The fibers which make up the **dorsal** aspect of the **stria terminalis** bundle effect rather widespread connections with hypothalamic and parolfactory areas. Cell bodies in the **medial** and **cortical** nuclei of the **amygdala** give rise to the fibers which course through the dorsal stria terminalis to the region of the anterior commissure. At this point, the fiber bundle splits into four components:

1. **Retrocommissural component.** This component courses ventrally through a region just posterior to the anterior commissure and terminates heavily in the **bed nucleus** of the **stria terminalis** and the **preoptic** region. These two regions of termination are continuous with each other.

2. **Commissural component.** A few fibers traverse through a posterior segment of the **anterior commissure** to terminate in the contralateral **bed nucleus** of the **stria terminalis** as well as the **contralateral cortical** and **medial** nuclei of the amygdala. This appears to be the only crossed component of the stria terminalis.

3. **Parolfactory component.** This component has a precommissural projection path and terminates diffusely in the ventral aspect of the **lateral septal nucleus,** in the **accumbens nucleus,** and in the **olfactory tubercle.** This rather limited projection to the lateral septum is the only association of the stria terminalis and the septal region, even though the gross appearance of this fiber bundle would suggest a major amygdaloseptal association pathway.

4. **Hypothalamic component.** These fibers are in close association with the fibers of the parolfactory division as they course over the anterodorsal aspect of the anterior commissure, but they then turn ventrally and terminate in the **medial preoptic** region and the **ventromedial hypothalamic nucleus.** The termination in the latter nucleus is rather interesting in that the projection is primarily to the outer surface of the nucleus, giving a "doughnut" type of appearance to the nucleus in both sagittal and coronal sections.

A summary of these projections is shown in Figure 7–2.

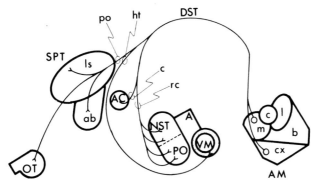

Fig. 7-2. Summary of the projections of the dorsal component of the stria terminalis (DST). AM = amygdala (cx = cortical nucleus, m = medial nucleus, c = central nucleus, l = lateral nucleus, b = basal nucleus), po = parolfactory component (ls = lateral septum, ab = accumbens nucleus, OT = olfactory tubercle), ht = hypothalamic component (VM = ventromedial hypothalamus), c = commissural component (AC = anterior commissure), rc = retrocommissural component (NST = nucleus of the stria terminalis, PO = preoptic region).

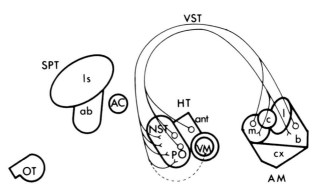

Fig. 7-3. Summary of the projections of the ventral component of the stria terminalis (VST). NST = nucleus of the stria terminalis, PO = preoptic area, ant = anterior regions of the hypothalamus (HT), AM = amygdala (cx = cortical nucleus, m = medial nucleus, c = central nucleus, l = lateral nucleus, b = basal nucleus).

VENTRAL COMPONENT OF STRIA TERMINALIS

The fibers which travel in the **ventral** aspect of the **stria terminalis** show a somewhat different origin within the amygdala and a more restricted pattern of projection. The cells which give rise to these fibers are located in the **medial** and **basolateral** nuclei of the **amygdala.** The fibers from these cells follow the stria terminalis and terminate **postcommissurally** in the **bed nucleus** of the **stria terminalis** and in the **preoptic nucleus.** A few fibers go beyond the preoptic region to terminate throughout the core of the **ventromedial hypothalamic nucleus,** as well as to the ventral and medial premammillary nuclei.

In addition to these projections from the amygdala to the hypothalamus, there are also reciprocal projections which arise from cells in the **anterior hypothalamus, preoptic region,** and the **bed nucleus** of the **stria terminalis** and terminate in the amygdala.

A summary of these projections is shown in Figure 7–3.

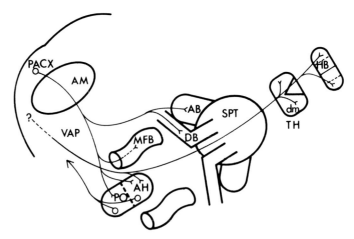

Fig. 7-4. Summary of the projections of the ventral amygdalofugal pathway (VAP) or the amygdalopyriform association bundle. PACX = periamygdaloid cortex, AM = amygdala, PO = preoptic area, AH = anterior hypothalamus, MFB = medial forebrain bundle, DB = diagonal band, AB = accumbens nucleus, SPT = septal region, dm = dorsomedial nucleus of the thalamus (TH), HB = habenula.

THE VENTRAL AMYGDALOFUGAL PATHWAY

77

STRIA TERMINALIS,
VENTRAL
AMYGDALOID
PATHWAYS,
AND AMYGDALOID
CONNECTIONS

Although the stria terminalis is the most obvious pathway connecting the amygdala to other structures, there is also a more diffuse (albeit more direct) pathway which courses along the ventral surface of the brain. The precise origins of this pathway have not been defined; although it is known that a large proportion of these fibers arises from cells in the **periamygdaloid cortex,** there is some question as to whether cells from the **basolateral amygdala** may also contribute. These fibers course medially and anteriorly to terminate widely in the lateral portion of the **preoptic nucleus,** the **accumbens nucleus,** the **diagonal band,** the **anterior hypothalamus,** and to more posterior locations via the **medial forebrain bundle.**

Fibers which arise from cells in the **preoptic nucleus** and the **anterior hypothalamus** form reciprocal connections with the amygdala. These reciprocating connections make the term ventral amygdalo**fugal** pathway something of a misnomer; it may be more appropriate to use Johnston's (1923) terminology, the **amygdalopyriform association bundle.**

Additional fibers of unknown origin within the amygdala follow a similar course to the preoptic region but then turn dorsally and project bilaterally to the **dorsomedial** and **habenular** nuclei of the thalamus.

A summary of these projections is shown in Figure 7–4.

OLFACTORY CONNECTIONS

Unlike many other regions of the so-called ''rhinencephalon,'' the amygdala does, in fact, have some rather substantial connections with the olfactory system. Fibers arising from the **olfactory bulb** project through the **lateral olfactory tract** and terminate in the

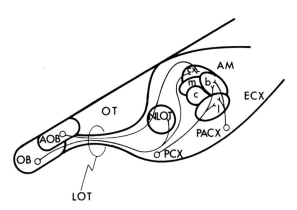

Fig. 7-5. Interconnections between the olfactory system and the amygdala. OB = olfactory bulb, AOB = accessory olfactory bulb, LOT = lateral olfactory tract, OT = olfactory tubercle, NLOT = nucleus of the lateral olfactory tract, PCX = pyriform cortex, PACX = periamygdaloid cortex, ECX = entorhinal cortex, AM = amygdala (cx = cortical nucleus, m = medial nucleus, b = basal nucleus, c = central nucleus, l = lateral nucleus).

anterior region of the **cortical amygdaloid nucleus** and in the **nucleus** of the **lateral olfactory tract.**

Fibers arising from the **accessory olfactory bulb** also project via the **lateral olfactory tract** but terminate in the posterior region of the **cortical nucleus.**

In addition to these primary olfactory connections, there are also projections which arise from cells in the **prepyriform** and **periamygdaloid cortex** and terminate in the **lateral** and **basal** nuclei of the amygdala.

A summary of these connections is shown in Figure 7–5.

SUMMARY

The amygdala is a structurally complicated set of nuclei that lies interposed between several major aspects of the basal forebrain. These nuclei have access to sensory information via rather direct interconnections with both the primary olfactory system and the accessory (vomeronasal) olfactory system. The fibers of the stria terminalis and the ventral projections interconnect the amygdala with structures extending from the base of the septum throughout the hypothalamus and preoptic region—structures that have access to higher-order olfactory and visceral input. Given these relationships with the hypothalamic and parolfactory regions, it seems likely that the amygdala will prove to be an important structure with respect to the olfactory system, sexual behavior, emotional behavior, and other behaviors that require interactions between olfactory and visceral information.

The Medial Forebrain Bundle and Related Hypothalamic Connections

8

INTRODUCTION

The medial forebrain bundle is a long, loosely textured fiber system which interconnects a variety of structures of the limbic and olfactory forebrain with the hypothalamus and the midbrain tegmentum. The parasagittal section reproduced in Figure 8–1 shows the major body of this rather massive fiber system as it passes caudally from the level of the anterior commissure to the posterior borders of the mammillary complex. As will be seen later, the more anterior and posterior projections of this system are somewhat more diffuse, and the various components of this system must be considered separately. Figure 8–2 shows this bundle of fibers in cross section at the level of the optic chiasm. At this level, and in fact throughout the system, the fibers are not seen as a compact bundle but rather are interspersed among cell bodies; in this particular instance, the cell bodies are those of the lateral hypothalamic nucleus.

Virtually all of the connections formed by the medial forebrain bundle are reciprocal in nature, i.e., the fiber projections are both ascending and descending. It should be noted, however, that the descending portion of the system is considerably larger than the ascending portion. Additionally, there is some degree of asymmetry in the connections formed by the ascending and descending components of the system. Accordingly, these two components will be considered separately.

Detailed descriptions may be found in technical articles by Gurdjian (1927), Loo (1930), Heimer and Nauta (1969), Nauta and Haymaker (in Haymaker, Anderson, & Nauta, 1969), and Leonard Scott (1971).

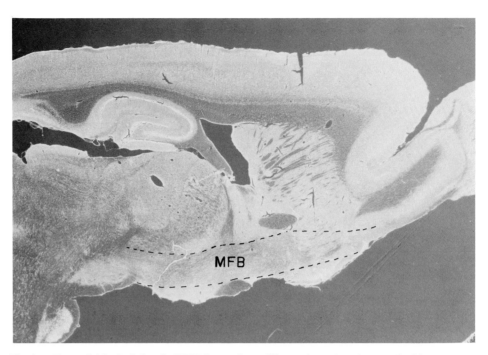

Fig. 8-1. The medial forebrain bundle (MFB) forms a long, diffuse pathway throughout much of the anteroposterior extent of the brain.

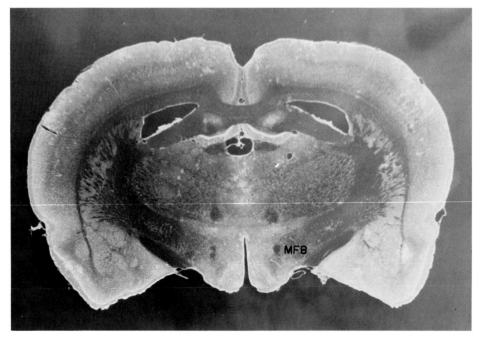

Fig. 8-2. The medial forebrain bundle (MFB) is shown in cross section as a somewhat diffuse bundle of fibers.

DESCENDING FIBERS OF THE MEDIAL FOREBRAIN BUNDLE

The major contribution to the descending portion of the medial forebrain bundle arises in the **septohippocampal** complex. Cell bodies from the posterior portion of **area CA 1** and from **areas CA 3** and **CA 4** of the hippocampus give rise to fibers which pass through the **precommissural** component of the **fornix** to terminate or to pass through virtually all aspects of the **septal area.** The fibers-in-passing from the fornix combine with fibers arising from the various septal nuclei to form an extensive descending system called the **septohypothalamic tract** (sometimes referred to as "Zuckerkandl's Riechbündl"). These fibers are in close association with the fibers of the diagonal band, lying just lateral to this system. A better appreciation of the mass of this system can be gained by viewing these fibers in the parasagittal plane, which reveals this fiber system descending along the entire anterodorsal extent of the septum. It should also be noted that some fibers from the postcommissural division of the stria terminalis may join these fibers en route to the medial forebrain bundle (see Fig. 8–3).

A second major source of fibers entering the descending medial forebrain bundle is the olfactory system (see Fig. 8–4). Cell bodies in the **anterior olfactory nucleus** and in the olfactory tubercle give rise to fibers which form the most anterior division of the medial forebrain bundle.

The details of the remainder of the descending system are not clearly defined, but it is known that fibers arise in the basal portion of the **caudate-putamen,** in the **pyriform cortex,** and in the **orbitofrontal cortex.**

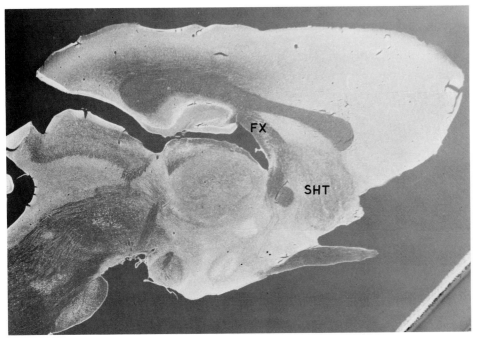

Fig. 8-3. The septohypothalamic tract forms a broad band of fibers collected from the fornix and septum and descending to the hypothalamus. SHT = septohypothalamic tract, FX = fornix.

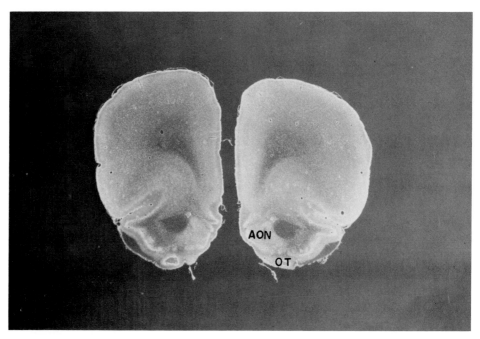

Fig. 8-4. The anterior olfactory nucleus and the olfactory tubercle give rise to fibers that form the anterior-most portions of the medial forebrain bundle. AON = anterior olfactory nucleus, OT = olfactory tubercle.

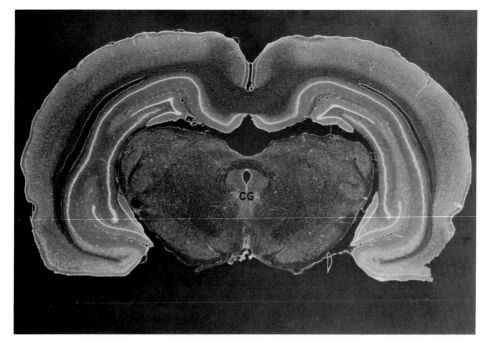

Fig. 8-5. The medial forebrain bundle projects to the central gray and the midbrain tegmental areas ventral to this region. CG = central gray.

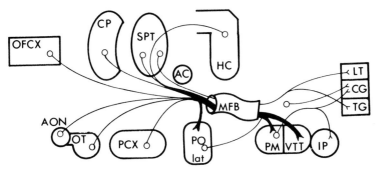

Fig. 8-6. Summary of the descending projections of the medial forebrain bundle (MFB). OFCX = orbitofrontal cortex, CP = caudate-putamen, SPT = septum, AC = anterior commissure, HC = hippocampus, AON = anterior olfactory nucleus, OT = olfactory tubercle, PCX = pyriform cortex, PO = preoptic region (lat = lateral), PM = premammillary nucleus, VTT = ventral tegmental area of Tsai, IP = interpeduncular nucleus, LT = lateral tegmentum, CG = central gray, TG = tegmentum.

All of the subdivisions that have been outlined converge at the level of the **preoptic nucleus** to form the body of the medial forebrain bundle. Because of this convergence of fibers, the medial forebrain bundle contains more fibers at this level than at any other point along its anterodorsal extent.

Many of the fibers that converge to form the medial forebrain bundle terminate in the **lateral preoptic nucleus** and in the **lateral hypothalamic area.** However, some of these fibers continue caudally, joined by fibers arising from the preoptic region, to terminate in

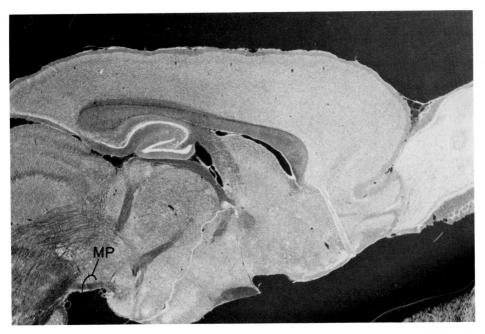

Fig. 8-7. Fibers from the midbrain tegmental area collect in the mammillary peduncle and the medial forebrain bundle. MP = mammillary peduncle.

the medial aspects of the **premammillary nucleus** and the **ventral tegmental area of Tsai.** The fibers which do not terminate in these structures are joined by fibers arising primarily from the mammillary complex and continue even further caudally to terminate rather diffusely in the **interpeduncular nucleus, the midbrain tegmentum,** and the **central gray.** (At this level, the projections are diffuse and the medial forebrain bundle is no longer seen as a discrete structure.) Although little is known about the details of this projection, there is some evidence that fibers arising from the septum may terminate somewhat more laterally than those arising from other sources and that the fibers arising from the lateral regions of the mammillary complex may project almost entirely to the central gray. Figure 8–5 shows the region to which many of these fibers project.

To summarize, fibers are collected from a wide variety of structures of the limbic and olfactory forebrain to form the medial forebrain bundle, which then forms synaptic connections along various levels of the hypothalamus extending caudally into the midbrain. A summary of these connections is shown in Figure 8–6.

ASCENDING COMPONENT OF THE MEDIAL FOREBRAIN BUNDLE

The ascending component arises from the same set of midbrain tegmental structures to which the descending component projects. Again, the details of the system have not been worked out, although a substantial portion of the system appears to arise from the **dorsal** and **ventral tegmental nuclei** (of Gudden) and the immediately surrounding area. These fibers form the **mammillary peduncle,** which courses anteriorly to form many synapses within the mammillary complex (see Fig. 8–7). At this level, a substantial number of these fibers join the medial forebrain bundle and project anteriorly to the **lateral hypothalamus,** the **lateral preoptic area,** and the nuclei of the **medial septum** and **diagonal band.** A few fibers may project into the **olfactory tubercle.** In addition to fibers arising in the midbrain tegmental region, there is also a component of fibers which originates in the **lateral hypothalamus** and projects to the **lateral septum.** These latter

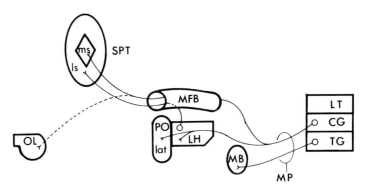

Fig. 8-8. Summary of the ascending component of the medial forebrain bundle (MFB). LT = lateral tegmentum, CG = central gray, TG = tegmentum, MP = mammillary peduncle, MB = mammillary body, LH = lateral hypothalamus, PO = preoptic region (lat = lateral), SPT = septum (ls = lateral septum, ms = medial septum), OL = olfactory structures.

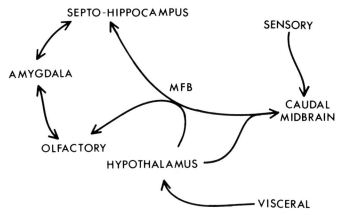

Fig. 8-9. An overview of the relationship of the medial forebrain bundle (MFB) to other brain systems.

fibers are considerably smaller in diameter than those midbrain fibers that project into the medial septum.

A summary of these connections is shown in Figure 8–8.

SUMMARY

Although it can always be considered somewhat myopic to consider a structure or a fiber system alone, rather than in relationship to other structures, this is particularly true in the case of the medial forebrain bundle. The structures of the forebrain are interconnected with each other via a number of different pathways and have access, albeit indirect in some cases, to a variety of sensory and visceral information. All of these structures contribute to the endocrine, autonomic, and motor outflow of the brain. When viewed in this perspective, the potential importance of the medial forebrain bundle, which interconnects these structures, is difficult to overemphasize. An overview of the position of the medial forebrain bundle with respect to other structures and systems is shown in Figure 8–9.

The Lateral Olfactory Tract, the Anterior Commissure, and Other Olfactory Connections

9

INTRODUCTION

Although all complex organisms utilize multisensory input to monitor the external environment, each species appears to have one system which is predominantly used. For man and most avian species, the dominant sensory system is vision. For rats and many other species of rodents, the dominant sensory system is olfaction. It is necessary to consider the olfactory system in some detail not only because it represents the primary source of sensory input for the rat, but also because of its close interrelationship with the structures of the limbic system; the notion that the primary function of the limbic system (rhinencephalon) was to process olfactory information is also of historical importance (cf. Chapter 1 and Brodal, 1947).

Although a great deal of information has been collected regarding the ultrastructure of the olfactory receptors, for the purposes of the present treatment, these structural characteristics will receive only a cursory review. The primary emphasis will be on the neuroanatomical connections.

Many of the central connections to be described have been presented in detail in excellent technical articles by Gurdjian (1925), Brodal (1948), Allison (1953), Powell, Cowan, & Raisman (1965), Price (1969), Land, Eager, & Shepherd (1970), and Raisman (1972).

OLFACTORY RECEPTION

The nose is an exquisitely sensitive chemical detection system which is designed to pick up airborne chemicals, dissolve them in the secretions of the nasal mucosae, and send information to the central nervous system regarding the nature of these chemicals. The impressive abilities of some organisms to detect odors are legendary: The bloodhound, for example, apparently can detect the presence of an individual human's odor which has passed through a thick leather sole of a shoe several hours earlier. Similarly, certain species of moths can detect a potential mate at distances of up to two miles on the basis of a specific odor cue known as a pheromone. Even the human nose—which has been battered by millenia of reduced evolutionary selection pressure, centuries of mucosal-parching heating systems, and decades of exposure to industrial waste products—has maintained a remarkable ability to detect airborne chemicals. A class of compounds called mercaptans, the most notable of which cause the odor of a skunk, can be detected under conditions in which as few as eight molecules of the substance enter the nose (cf. De Vries & Stuiver, 1959).

The olfactory receptor cells and supporting cells are located in the nasal mucosae. Typically, these receptors are concentrated in the relatively deep recesses of the olfactory sinuses so that sniffing must occur in order to produce eddy currents, thereby gaining maximal exposure of the airborne substance to the receptors.

In addition to these olfactory receptors, the rat also has specialized receptors in the **vomeronasal (Jacobson's) organ** that may respond to a combination of taste and olfactory stimuli. As will be shown, the central projection from this organ shares many of the same anatomical pathways as are involved in the main olfactory system.

The actual chemically specific receptor units are located on the olfactory cilia, which protrude from the surface of the mucosa and are bathed in a fluid secreted by the mucosal lining. In man, there are some 60 million receptors squeezed into an area about the size of the end of one's nose. The protruding cilia increase the functional area dramatically, perhaps to as much as several times that of the outer body surface (Milner, 1970). The fibers which leave the base of the receptive units are quite small, less than $0.2\ \mu$ in diameter, and are collected into tiny bundles which pass through holes in the sievelike structure of the overlying bone (**cribriform plate**) to reach the surface of the olfactory bulb. Thus the olfactory nerve is made up of extremely small fibers, which are only a few millimeters in length and which are embedded within a bony plate deep within the skull.

After passing through the cribriform plate, the fibers of the olfactory nerve cover the anterior surface of the olfactory bulbs and make complicated connections within the bulbs. The synaptic connections of these filaments are not evenly distributed but, rather, form small round bodies known as the **olfactory glomeruli.** These glomeruli represent connections of olfactory nerve fibers with dendrites of mitral cells, tufted cells, and granular cells (Allison, 1953; Minckler, 1972). Located further within the bulb are additional connections within the granular layers. At least several hundred olfactory receptors converge upon each tufted cell or mitral cell. This type of complex, converging interconnection typifies systems that are highly sensitive but which adapt readily (see Fig. 9–1).

The cross-sectional view of the olfactory bulb shown in Figure 9–2 indicates one of the major characteristics of this structure, namely, that the cell bodies and fibers which make up the bulb are arranged in concentric layers, suggesting a highly organized system of interconnections. The remainder of this chapter will be devoted to a description of the central nervous system connections of the olfactory system, particularly as they relate to the limbic system.

89

LATERAL
OLFACTORY TRACT,
ANTERIOR
COMMISSURE, AND
OTHER OLFACTORY
CONNECTIONS

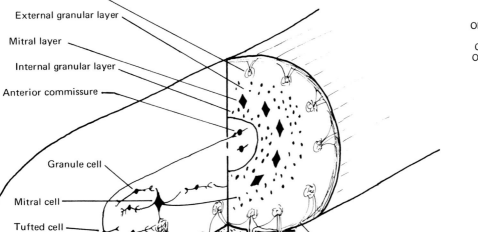

Glomerular layer

External granular layer

Mitral layer

Internal granular layer

Anterior commissure

Granule cell

Mitral cell

Tufted cell

Glomerulus

Nerve filaments

Olfactory receptors

Cribriform plate

Fig. 9-1. Schematic diagram of the relationships among various olfactory structures.

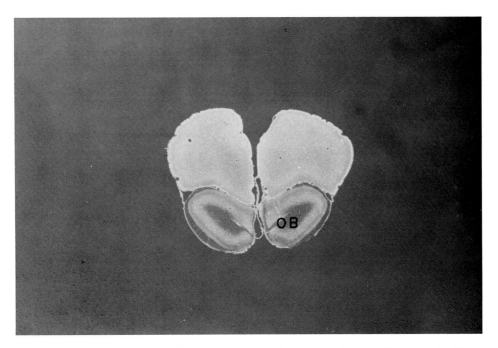

OB

Fig. 9-2. Cross section through the olfactory bulbs showing the concentric layers of fibers and cells. OB = olfactory bulbs.

THE CENTRAL OLFACTORY CONNECTIONS

There are two major fiber systems which are easily discernible through gross inspection of the brain. One of these is the **intermediate olfactory tract,** which arises from axons of tufted cells and travels posteriorly through the center of the **olfactory bulb** to become the **anterior commissure** (which crosses the midline in the septal region just below the genu of the corpus callosum). In horizontal sections, these fibers form a broad, horseshoe-shaped arc across the midline (see, e.g., Fig. 4–14).

The second major fiber system is the **lateral olfactory tract,** which arises from mitral cell axons and courses along the inferior and lateral surface of the bulbs and continues posteriorly to the level of the amygdala (see Chapter 4).

The Anterior Commissure

As the name implies, the anterior commissure has long been considered to be a commissural system that provides point-to-point interconnections between homotopic regions of the two olfactory bulbs. More recent evidence (e.g., Powell *et al.,* 1965) suggests that this view is not entirely correct: The mitral cell bodies of the olfactory bulb per se do not give rise to the fibers of the anterior commissure but rather project to the **anterior olfactory nucleus.** This nucleus, in turn, contributes the fibers of the anterior commissure; these fibers cross the midline and return in the contralateral limb of the commissure, at which point the projection splits into a **dorsal component** and a **rostral component.** The dorsal component turns upward to terminate in the **accessory olfactory bulb,** which lies on the dorsal surface of the main bulb. The rostral component projects further anteriorly and terminates in the **anterior olfactory nucleus** and the main **olfactory bulb.** These latter olfactory bulb connections are primarily in the dendrites of the **internal granular cells** surrounding the intermediate olfactory tract. Because of the asymmetry of the origins and terminations of this fiber system, it is, strictly speaking, not a commissural system but rather a **crossed projection system** (see Fig. 9–3).

Although the major portion of the anterior commissure is a crossed system, there is also a **deep ipsilateral projection** of the anterior commissure which essentially duplicates

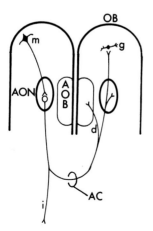

Fig. 9-3. Summary of the connections of the anterior limb of the anterior commissure. AC = anterior commissure (i = ipsilateral component, d = dorsal component), OB = olfactory bulb (m = mitral cells, g = granule cells), AOB = accessory bulbs, AON = anterior olfactory nucleus.

the projection pathway of the lateral olfactory tract (to be described). The major difference is that these fibers tend to terminate on the deeper aspects of the cells involved, whereas the remaining fibers of the lateral olfactory tract tend to terminate on the apical dendrites.

Thus far, only the **anterior limb** of the anterior commissure has been described. As has been previously indicated (cf. Fig. 4–14), these fibers are joined as they cross the midline by the **intertemporal component,** consisting of crossed projections from the **pyriform cortex,** and by fibers from the **stria terminalis;** the significance, if any, of these connections with respect to olfaction is unknown.

91

LATERAL
OLFACTORY TRACT,
ANTERIOR
COMMISSURE, AND
OTHER OLFACTORY
CONNECTIONS

The Lateral Olfactory Tract

Most of the fibers of the lateral olfactory tract are the long axons of the **mitral cells** of the olfactory bulb. These fibers course posteriorly along the base of the brain to terminate in the **pyriform cortex,** the **olfactory tubercle,** the **nucleus of the lateral olfactory tract,** and the **anterior olfactory nucleus.**

Fibers arising from the **olfactory tubercle** and **pyriform cortex** also project to the lateral regions of the hypothalamus and preoptic region via both the **medial forebrain bundle** and the **lateral olfactory tract.** A few of these fibers may course as far posteriorly as the cortical nucleus of the amygdala.

The lateral olfactory tract also contains fibers arising from the cortical regions medial to this tract. These fibers terminate in the **posterior hypothalamus** and in the small **gemini nuclei,** located just laterally to the mammillothalamic tract.

The **pyriform cortex** not only receives a large number of olfactory fibers but also serves as a sort of relay between the primary olfactory structures and a rather widely distributed set of secondary and tertiary structures. Fibers arising from cells in the **anterior** portion of the pyriform cortex project **caudally** along two routes: (1) a superficial route which terminates in the **posterior** regions of the **pyriform cortex** and in the **entorhinal cortex** and (2) a deep route which projects to the deeper regions of the pyriform and entorhinal cortices as well as to the **basal** and **lateral amygdaloid nuclei.** Neither of these projections reaches the hippocampus or the subiculum.

Fibers arising from both the anterior and posterior portions of the pyriform cortex form a **medial projection** system that terminates in the **olfactory tubercle,** the **anterior subcallosal cortex,** the **nucleus of the diagonal band** (from anterior regions only), and the **lateral preoptic nucleus.**

Although most of the fibers of the lateral olfactory tract are **centripetal** (projecting into the central nervous system), there is also a smaller component of **centrifugal** fibers which conduct central influences out to the bulb. The bulk of these fibers arise from the **pyriform cortex** and **olfactory tubercle** to form a polysynaptic pathway connecting these structures to the **anterior olfactory nucleus** and the **internal granular cells** of the olfactory bulb. These latter structures also receive fibers arising from the nucleus of the horizontal limb of the **diagonal band.**

As shown in the summary diagram of Figure 9–4, the olfactory system terminates heavily in a broad field that extends through the entire anterodorsal extent of the lateral preoptic and hypothalamic regions, the olfactory tubercle, the pyriform cortex, and portions of the amygdala. From these structures, there are heavy projections of other limbic system structures as well as reciprocal connections within the olfactory system.

The Vomeronasal System

As mentioned before, a rather specialized structure located in the nasal cavity of the rat contributes to the olfactory tract (see Fig. 9–5). These fibers synapse with the **mitral cells** of the **accessory olfactory bulb** in the same manner as the main olfactory fibers synapse within the main olfactory bulb. These mitral cells give rise to fibers that course caudally via the **lateral olfactory tract** to terminate in the posterior regions of the **cortical amygdaloid nucleus** and possibly in the medial nucleus. Fibers arising from these regions of the amygdala enter the **stria terminalis** and project to the **medial preoptic area** as well as the **ventromedial** nucleus of the **hypothalamus.** Some of these stria terminalis fibers apparently project rostrally to terminate on the **internal granule cells** of the accessory olfactory bulb, thereby completing a reciprocal circuit similar to that which exists for the main bulbs. The precise function of this system is not known.

SUMMARY

The olfactory system has been given special consideration in this chapter because of its historical importance with respect to the notion of a rhinencephalon, because of its importance in the behavioral repertoire of the rat, and because there are several aspects of its organization that make its relationship to the limbic system unique among the senses.

The organization of the olfactory receptor cells and the cells of the olfactory bulbs per se provide the anatomical substrate for an extremely sensitive chemical detection system. Not only is there a high degree of convergence (i.e., many receptors funneling into a single fiber), but there also appear to be recurrent collaterals that function as a positive feedback system to further enhance the original stimulus. There is a possibility for even

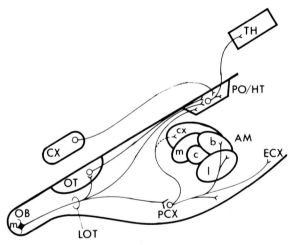

Fig. 9-4. Summary of the connections of the lateral olfactory tract (LOT). OB = olfactory bulb (m = mitral cell), OT = olfactory tubercle, CX = cortex, PCX = pyriform cortex, ECX = entorhinal cortex, AM = amygdala (cx = cortical nucleus, b = basal nucleus, c = central nucleus, m = medial nucleus, l = lateral nucleus), PO/HT = preoptic/hypothalamic region, TH = thalamus.

93

LATERAL
OLFACTORY TRACT,
ANTERIOR
COMMISSURE, AND
OTHER OLFACTORY
CONNECTIONS

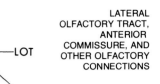

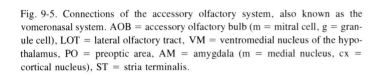

Fig. 9-5. Connections of the accessory olfactory system, also known as the vomeronasal system. AOB = accessory olfactory bulb (m = mitral cell, g = granule cell), LOT = lateral olfactory tract, VM = ventromedial nucleus of the hypothalamus, PO = preoptic area, AM = amygdala (m = medial nucleus, cx = cortical nucleus), ST = stria terminalis.

further integration of olfactory stimuli at the level of the olfactory bulbs and associated nuclei via the crossed projections of the anterior commissure.

Most of the fibers that arise in the olfactory bulbs project via the lateral olfactory tract to terminate in the pyriform cortex. Thus, the olfactory system is unlike any other sensory system in that it projects to a cortical region without first going through a thalamic relay. The cells of the pyriform cortex give rise to higher-order fibers that project to a variety of areas, including the amygdala, the entorhinal cortex, and a basal region extending from the lateral preoptic region along the entire lateral aspect of the hypothalamus. The lateral hypothalamic zone may have important functional roles in such things as endocrine function, consummatory behaviors, and behaviors that involve varying degrees of hormonal control. In addition to the projections from the pyriform cortex, the lateral hypothalamic region also receives fibers from another primitive cortical region, the hippocampus. Since the hippocampus has access to both higher-order olfactory information and information from other sensory systems, the possibility for integration at the hypothalamus seems likely. It should also be pointed out that the amygdala relays olfactory information to the medial aspects of the hypothalamus.

In addition to the interaction of the hippocampus and pyriform cortex at the hypothalamic level, both systems project to the thalamus, the hippocampus projecting to the anterior nuclei and the pyriform cortex to the dorsomedial nuclei. Here again, the possibility of interaction of olfactory information with that of other sensory systems is apparent.

Finally, it should be noted that both the hippocampal complex and the pyriform cortex project (directly and via the lateral preoptic region) to the lateral habenula. This projection provides yet another important avenue of interaction with the limbic system via the habenulo-interpenduncular route to the limbic midbrain regions. It should be apparent from the summary of the olfactory connections that the limbic system is ideally situated for the analysis of olfactory information. Thus, the discontinuation of the term "rhinencephalon" should imply only that this is not the exclusive function of the limbic system, rather than implying that the limbic system has little or no involvement in olfactory processing.

Cortical Extensions of the Limbic System

10

INTRODUCTION

The cortex of the rat forms a smooth, relatively thin mantle over most of the structures that have been discussed thus far. Because the cortex is smooth, rather than convoluted, as in the case of animals having a more highly developed brain, the cerebral hemispheres are termed **lissencephalic.** The conceptual subdivision of a smooth mantle of cortex involves some technical difficulties, because there are few landmarks that can be used. Consequently, many of the subdivisions that have been made are based either on the detailed cellular structure of the layered cortex or on the juxtaposition to more clearly defined subcortical structures. The details of categorizing areas of the cortex on the basis of cellular organization go beyond the scope of this text, so the descriptions that follow will emphasize boundaries with respect to available landmarks. In most cases, though, the delineations were originally made by the careful study of cellular organization. Most notable in these types of studies are the classic descriptions of Krieg (1946) and Rose and Woolsey (1948). Additional accounts of these cortical systems and their connections may be found in articles by Clark (1932), Clark and Boggon (1933), Lorente de Noʹ (1934), Abbie (1938), Krieg (1947), Domesick (1969), and Leonard (1969).

CINGULATE CORTEX

Topography

The cingulate cortex is a thin layer of cortical tissue that forms the walls of the longitudinal fissure. As shown in Figure 10–1, the cingulate cortex occupies the entire medial aspect of the hemisphere above the level of the corpus callosum. The cellular structure allows a distinction to be made between the **posterior cingulate cortex** (also called the **retrosplenial area**) and the **anterior cingulate cortex** (also called the **area infraradiata**). The cortical tissue extends somewhat below the level of the commissure both anterior to the genu and posterior to the splenium. (As will be indicated later, there is some feeling among more recent investigators that it would be more appropriate conceptually to include the anterior cingulate cortex as a part of the frontal cortex.)

A dorsal view of the brain reveals only a narrow band of cingulate cortex on either side of the midline. In other words, this structure shows only a very limited spread over the dorsal surface of the brain, being almost entirely concealed within the fold of the longitudinal fissure.

Connections of the Cingulate Cortex

An understanding of the connections of the cingulate cortex requires an appreciation of the general topography of the thalamic nuclei, which are rather closely interconnected with this region of the cortex. For the present purposes, the thalamic nuclei will be depicted in highly schematized form, and the reader is referred to Chapter 2 for descriptions of the three-dimensional characteristics of these nuclei.

As indicated in Figure 10–2, the anterior and posterior divisions of the cingulate cortex show differential projections to the thalamic nuclei. Fibers arising from the cell bodies of the **anterior cingulate gyrus** penetrate the corpus callosum to terminate in the **dorsomedial nucleus** of the **thalamus**. (It should be noted that the vast majority of the fibers of the corpus callosum course transversely, interconnecting the two hemispheres; many of the connections between cortical and subcortical regions pass through this thick band of fibers in numerous small bundles.) This anterior cingulate projection appears to be somewhat systematic in that the distribution of terminations within the dorsomedial nu-

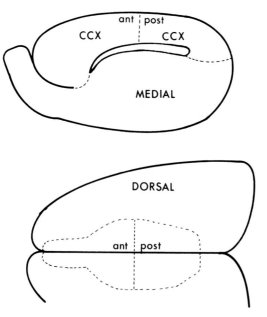

Fig. 10-1. Dorsal and medial sketches of the brain showing the approximate boundaries of the cingulate cortex (CCX) (ant = anterior division, post = posterior division).

cleus bear the same general spatial relationships as the cells of origin. There is also a smaller projection of fibers that originates in the most anterior portions of the cingulate cortex and travels below (rather than through) the corpus callosum to terminate in the **ventromedial nucleus** of the **thalamus.**

The **posterior cingulate gyrus** gives rise to fibers that course anteriorly along the dorsal surface of the corpus callosum in the **cingulum bundle.** Ultimately, these fibers turn ventrally and travel through the fibers of the corpus callosum to terminate primarily within the **anteroventral nucleus;** there are, however, some terminations in the dorsolateral nucleus as well. There may be some reciprocal fibers arising in the anteroventral nucleus and terminating in the posterior cingulate cortex, but these would appear to be small in number if they exist at all.

In addition to the connections with the thalamic nuclei, both the anterior and the posterior divisions of the cingulate cortex project to a variety of other subcortical areas. Included among these are the zona incerta, the caudate-putamen, the tegmentum, the superior colliculi, the pretectum, and the central gray. It must be emphasized that in the rat there is no evidence for terminations in the traditional limbic system structures such as the septum, amygdala, hypothalamus, and mammillary bodies. This lack of a close interrelationship with the limbic system draws into question the somewhat routine inclusion of the cingulate cortex as an integral part of the limbic system. But the cingulate gyrus has indirect access to traditional limbic system influences, and there is some convergence of limbic system and cingulate cortex influences in the midbrain (see Fig. 10–3).

FRONTAL CORTEX

Topography

The term "frontal cortex" must be used with some caution in the case of the rat. As indicated earlier, the delineation of various portions of the cortex is tedious because of the criteria that are used. This problem becomes even more difficult when an attempt is made to determine homologous regions between two or more different species. In man and other primates, the frontal cortex is characterized by large granule cells in the fourth layer of the cortex. This characteristic is not observed in rats and many other subprimates, a fact which could indicate that there are no homologous regions. But the cellular structure and organization are not the only criteria that can be used—another criterion is to determine

Fig. 10-2. Summary of the projections from the cingulate cortex. CCX = cingulate cortex (ant = anterior division, post = posterior division), TH = thalamus (ad = anterodorsal, dl = dorsolateral, am = anteromedial, dm = dorsomedial, av = anteroventral, vm = ventromedial), etc. = a variety of other subcortical areas (see text).

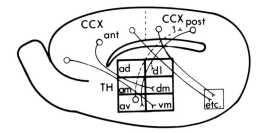

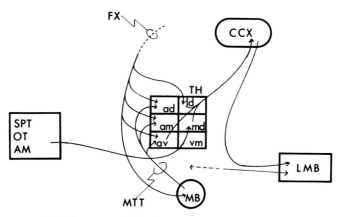

Fig. 10-3. Convergence of limbic system and cingulate cortex projections in the midbrain. SPT = septum, OT = olfactory tubercle, AM = amygdala, FX = fornix, TH = thalamus (ad = anterodorsal, am = anteromedial, ld = dorsolateral, md = dorsomedial, av = anteroventral, vm = ventromedial), CCX = cingulate cortex, MTT = mammillothalamic tract, MB = mammillary body, LMB = limbic midbrain.

the connections of a particular region and compare these connections with those of another species. When this approach is used, it appears that the rat does, in fact, possess a homologue to the frontal cortex in spite of the lack of similarity in the detailed cytoarchitecture (cf. Leonard, 1969).

Figure 10–4 indicates that the frontal cortex constitutes most of the surface of the anterior half of the brain, from a point near the midline laterally to the rhinal sulcus. The anterior region of the medial wall of the hemisphere is traditionally considered to be a part of the cingulate cortex.

Given this definition of the frontal cortex, this structure can be viewed as a sort of cup-shaped layer of tissue that encapsulates the anterior regions of the hemispheres, extending back to approximately the level of the genu of the corpus callosum along the

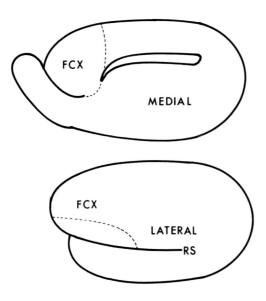

Fig. 10-4. Medial and lateral sketches of the brain showing the approximate boundaries of the frontal cortex (FCX). RS = rhinal sulcus.

medial aspect and more posteriorly to about the midportion of the hemisphere along the lateral aspects. For the purposes of describing connections from the frontal cortex, it is useful to designate a sulcal region (which is adjacent to the rhinal sulcus) and a medial region (which forms the wall of the anterior portion of the longitudinal fissure).

Connections of the Frontal Cortex

One of the major sources of fibers terminating in the frontal cortex is the dorsomedial nucleus of the thalamus, which contributes two somewhat distinct sets of fibers. Cell bodies in the **posterior** portion of the **dorsomedial nucleus** project laterally through the reticular nucleus of the thalamus and the caudate-putamen to enter the **internal capsule.** After entering the internal capsule, these fibers disperse rather widely to terminate along the **sulcal region** of the frontal cortex.

The second contribution arises from the **anterior** portion of the **dorsomedial nucleus** and follows a somewhat similar course, except that many of the fibers join the **cingulum** at the level of the genu of the corpus callosum and then terminate in the **ventral** and **medial** aspects of the frontal poles. In both of these systems, there are apparently some terminations in the **reticular nucleus** of the thalamus and in the **caudate-putamen.**

Another major thalamic contribution to the frontal cortex arises in the **anteromedial nucleus.** Cell bodies from this region give rise to fibers that terminate along the **medial wall** of the frontal cortex.

Finally, there are a few fibers that arise from cells in the **ventromedial nucleus** of the **thalamus** and project to a small region along the deepest aspect of the rhinal sulcus, immediately adjacent to the pyriform cortex.

A summary of these different connections of the frontal cortex is shown in Figure 10–5.

The efferent connections of the medial and sulcal portions of the frontal cortex exhibit different patterns of termination. Fibers that arise from cell bodies in the **medial aspects** of the frontal cortex descend through the corpus callosum (some fibers join the

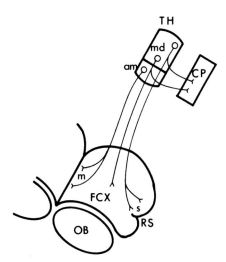

Fig. 10-5. Summary of afferent projections to the frontal cortex. TH = thalamus (md = dorsomedial, am = anteromedial), CP = caudate-putamen, m = medial division of frontal cortex (FCX), s = sulcal region of frontal cortex, RS = rhinal sulcus.

corpus callosum and cross to the contralateral side) and travel through the caudate-putamen in small bundles before entering the **external capsule.** The fibers are then distributed broadly to subcortical structures including the **olfactory tubercle, thalamus, hypothalamus,** and **midbrain tegmentum.**

Fibers that arise from the **sulcal region** of the frontal cortex also descend through the corpus callosum, caudate-putamen, and external capsule but then are distributed to other regions via somewhat different pathways. In addition to rather substantial projections to the **midline thalamic nuclei** (adjacent to the ventricle), there are projections to the **lateral** regions of the midbrain tegmentum via the cerebral peduncle and to the **substantia innominata, olfactory tubercle,** and **rostral hypothalamus** via the medial forebrain bundle.

A summary of these efferent projections of the frontal cortex is shown in Figure 10–6.

In summary, the frontal cortex is interconnected with a variety of subcortical structures that are indirectly related to the limbic system, but there are few connections with traditional limbic system structures. Thus, the frontal cortex, either narrowly or broadly defined, is similar to the cingulate cortex in that there is considerable reason to suspect a somewhat indirect interaction with the limbic system, via mutual interconnections to the thalamus, hypothalamus, and midbrain.

THE ENTORHINAL CORTEX

Topography

The entorhinal cortex covers the most posterior and ventral aspects of the hemispheres (see Fig. 10–7). The medial aspect of the brain shows only a thin band of the entorhinal cortex juxtaposed with the anterior portion of the cerebellum. Laterally, the

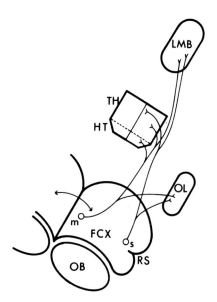

Fig. 10-6. Summary of the efferent projections from the frontal cortex. RS = rhinal sulcus, m = medial region of frontal cortex (FCX), s = sulcal region on frontal cortex, OL = olfactory structures, HT = hypothalamus, TH = thalamus, LMB = limbic midbrain.

entorhinal cortex is located beneath the posterior portion of the rhinal sulcus and is, accordingly, a part of the general rhinal cortex (the prefix "ento-" means within). Because of the nature of the connections to be discussed, it is useful to designate the medial and lateral aspects of this region. As indicated in horizontal sections, the medial portion lies immediately posterior to the hippocampal complex, whereas the lateral portion lies laterally to these structures. The entire entorhinal cortex lies posterior to the level of the amygdaloid complex, which allows a distinction to be made between the periamygdaloid cortex and the entorhinal cortex.

Connections of the Entorhinal Cortex

The connections of the entorhinal cortex have only recently been determined in detail. Although it has long been known that the entorhinal area contributes fibers to the hippocampus, the precise nature of this contribution and the presence of reciprocal connections were determined only through modern staining techniques. The entorhinal cortex is separated from the hippocampus by the subiculum and the presubiculum, so any fiber connections between the hippocampus and the entorhinal cortex must penetrate or perfo-

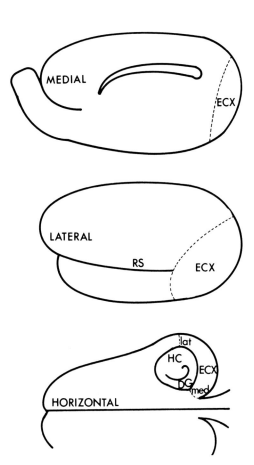

Fig. 10-7. Medial, lateral, and horizontal sketches of the brain showing the approximate outline of the entorhinal cortex (ECX) (med = medial division, lat = lateral division), HC = hippocampus, DG = dentate gyrus, RS = rhinal sulcus.

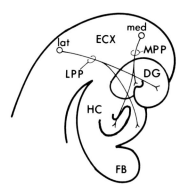

Fig. 10-8. Summary of the projections of the entorhinal cortex via the perforant pathways. ECX = entorhinal cortex (med = medial division, lat = lateral division), MPP = medial perforant pathway, LPP = lateral perforant pathway, DG = dentate gyrus, HC = hippocampus, FB = fimbria.

rate these cortical regions. Accordingly, these fibers have been termed the **perforant pathways,** which can be subdivided into medial and lateral divisions (see Fig. 10–8).

The **medial entorhinal area** projects rather directly to the hippocampus via the **medial perforant pathway.** Specifically, the fibers terminate in the middle of the molecular layer of the **dentate gyrus** and in the deep aspects of **area CA 3** of the **hippocampus.**

The lateral entorhinal cortex gives rise to fibers that form the **lateral perforant pathway** and terminate in the superficial molecular layer of the **dentate gyrus** and the superficial aspects of **area CA 3** of the **hippocampus.**

Reciprocal connections from the hippocampus to the entorhinal cortex arise from **area CA 3** and are distributed topographically to the entorhinal cortex along a dorsoventral plane (Hjorth-Simonsen, 1971), i.e., the most ventral aspects of the hippocampus project to the most ventral aspects of the entorhinal cortex while more dorsally located regions project to more dorsally located regions of the entorhinal cortex (see Fig. 10–9).

The connections of the entorhinal cortex suggest a major role of the structure in limbic system functions. It is essentially a cortical extension of the largest and structurally most complex component of the limbic system—the hippocampus. In the discussion of the fornix system in Chapter 3, it was noted that this system of fibers provides interconnections between a septohippocampal complex and various thalamic, hypothalamic, and midbrain regions. The highly systematic connections of the hippocampus and entorhinal cortex will probably result, eventually, in the designation of a septo-hippocampal-entorhinal complex.

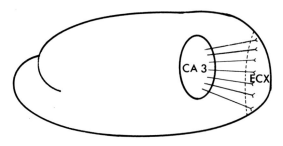

Fig. 10-9. Summary of the topographic projection of the hippocampus to the entorhinal cortex (ECX).

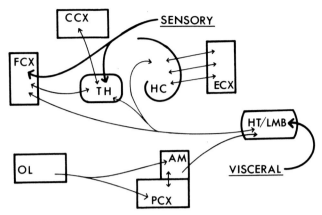

Fig. 10-10. An overview of the relationship of the various cortical regions to the limbic system and other aspects of the brain. FCX = frontal cortex, CCX = cingulate cortex, TH = thalamus, HC = hippocampus, ECX = entorhinal cortex, OL = olfactory structures, AM = amygdala, PCX = pyriform cortex, HT/LMB = hypothalamus/limbic midbrain.

THE PYRIFORM CORTEX

The pyriform cortex is intimately involved with the olfactory system and the amygdala. The reader is referred to the appropriate sections of Chapters 7 and 9 for a discussion of the topography and connections of this cortical region.

SUMMARY

In summary, there are four major subdivisions of the cortical mantel that have been implicated in limbic system circuitry.

The **cingulate cortex** was included in Papez' (1937) early theoretical paper as a major component of the so-called visceral brain. More recent evidence suggests a somewhat less direct role of this structure.

The **entorhinal cortex** is unquestionably linked to the limbic system, recent studies having shown a highly organized system of interconnections with the hippocampus. Interestingly, this structure was not even mentioned in Papez' (1937) classical treatise on the limbic system.

The **pyriform cortex** is interconnected with both the olfactory system and the amygdala. As such, it is the only cortical region of the limbic system that is directly involved in olfaction.

The **frontal cortex,** as traditionally defined, has not evolved to much extent in the rat brain. This oversight of evolution has been partially adjusted for by recent neuroanatomists who have enlarged the designation of the frontal cortex on the basis of anatomical connections. As will be noted in the final chapter, the recent demonstration of multisensory projections to the frontal cortex (cf. Powell, 1973) has suggested some new interpretations of the functional role of the frontal cortex.

A summary of the general relationship of these cortical regions is shown in Figure 10–10.

Histochemical Mapping of the Limbic System

11

INTRODUCTION

One of the fundamental principles characterizing all histological procedures is selectivity. Although the ultimate goal in staining of the central nervous system is to provide a description of all the interconnections of the brain, each particular method gains its power from the property of selectively staining only certain aspects of the central nervous system. In some cases, such as the original Golgi method, the stain impregnates the entire cell and its processes, but, for reasons that are not understood, the method affects only about 5% of the total population of cells. If this were not the case, the stain would not have been useful to Golgi because of the limitations in producing thin slices of tissue—thick sections in which all the cells are stained would be nearly opaque, obscuring any cellular detail.

More recently developed procedures stain specific structures, i.e., the cell body or fibers, degenerating fibers, fibers that contain a certain neurotransmitter, or fibers that have been pretreated with a compound that is incorporated into the metabolic machinery of the cell (see Chapter 2 for examples). In each instance, the selectivity of the technique has revealed certain aspects of nervous system organization that cannot be observed using other procedures.

One of the most promising approaches to the study of brain circuitry has been the development of histochemical processes that make use of the presumed chemical specificity of neurons. Although few substances unequivocally meet the criteria defining a central neurotransmitter (cf. Goodman & Gilman, 1965), there are a number of putative neurotransmitters that are likely to be involved in central nervous system functions. Among these are acetylcholine, serotonin, norepinephrine, and dopamine. Knowledge of the metabolic pathways specific to each proposed transmitter substance has allowed the development of staining procedures that interact with some unique aspect of each neurotransmitter system. This technique, therefore, makes it possible to stain a population of neurons in the central nervous system that contains a particular neurotransmitter substance. To the extent that a functional system may be organized on the basis of a common neurotransmitter, the ability to trace these pathways may reveal both the functional and the anatomical organization of the brain. The following summaries of recent histochemical findings will outline the chemical pathways that have been related to limbic system structures.

MONOAMINES

In the early 1960s, two separate lines of research were undertaken to investigate the distribution of central nervous system neurons that contain the monoamines which are believed to be neurotransmitters (norepinephrine, serotonin, and dopamine). A group of investigators in the United States observed that certain lesions of the brain stem and hypothalamic region resulted in a dramatic increase in sleeping time induced by anesthesia (Harvey, Heller, Moore, Hunt, & Roth, 1964). Based on these behavioral observations, it was predicted that the brain stem damage interfered with serotonergic systems, and a series of experiments was performed to determine the effects of these lesions on the chemical transmitter system. Whole-brain assays of serotonin levels revealed that lesions of the lateral hypothalamus or certain areas of the tegmentum produced a substantial reduction in brain serotonin levels, presumably as a result of the degeneration of serotonin-containing neurons (Moore & Heller, 1967; Moore, Wong, & Heller, 1965). Later studies showed that this decrease was rather specific and could be attributed primarily to a system that originated in the central gray region and traveled through the medial forebrain bundle (see Moore, 1970a for review). Additional chemical assays revealed that the medial forebrain bundle damage which reduced serotonin levels also reduced norepinephrine levels but that the midbrain central gray damage had little or no effect on the amount of norepinephrine (Heller & Moore, 1965). In both instances, the decrease in norepinephrine or serotonin levels occurred only in brain regions that were anterior to the point of damage. The data strongly suggest that these are primarily ascending systems which originate in different regions but are closely related within the medial forebrain bundle.

The second line of research was being undertaken in Sweden by a group of researchers using histochemical techniques. In 1962, Falck devised a histofluorescent technique for staining fibers that contain serotonin, dopamine, or norepinephrine. Some of the initial work revealed monoamine-containing cells in the midbrain regions, paralleling findings that damage to these areas is followed by a lowered level of monoamines. Andén, Dahlström, Fuxe, Larsson, Olsen, and Ungerstedt (1966) studied these systems in more detail by combining this new histofluorescent technique with either selective brain lesions or the administration of drugs that have known interactions with monoaminergic systems. On the basis of these experiments, they were able to outline the origins and projections of several different transmitter systems.

Although the data from these two groups of researchers are directly comparable in terms of the origin and distribution of the different fiber systems, there are differences in interpretation that exemplify the limitations of each approach. Heller and his associates (cf. Moore, 1970) suggest that the noradrenergic system is polysynaptic, having cell bodies not only in the midbrain, but also distributed throughout the medial forebrain bundle. This argument is based on the fact that the depletion of norepinephrine which would be expected if all the cells of origin were destroyed or if all the fibers within the medial forebrain bundle were transected is never complete. The Swedish group, on the other hand, argues that this system is monosynaptic with long fibers extending from cell bodies located in the midbrain. The resolution of this problem requires either a demonstration that long fibers course from the midbrain all the way to the cortex or, conversely, that there are cell bodies that form relays en route, perhaps in the medial forebrain bundle. Unfortunately, the fibers involved are small, and it has been virtually impossible to provide unequivocal support for either position. Given the rapid advances that are being made in neuroanatomical techniques, this issue will likely be settled within the next few years. Regardless of whether the monoamine depletion that follows midbrain lesions is the result of direct degeneration or transynaptic effects, the basic pathways and distribution of the fibers will probably need little modification from that which has been established using the currently available techniques. A series of reports by the Swedish investigators has provided most of the information regarding these pathways, the details of which may be found either in the original sources (cf. Ungerstedt, 1971; Carlsson, Falck, & Hillarp, 1962; Andén *et al.*, 1966; Dahlström & Fuxe, 1964) or in an excellent review and extension by Lindvall and Björklund (1974).

107

HISTOCHEMICAL
MAPPING
OF THE
LIMBIC
SYSTEM

The Noradrenergic Systems

The Dorsal Noradrenergic Bundle. The largest concentration of norepinephrine-containing cell bodies reported by Dahlström and Fuxe (1964) was in an area of the brain stem that they referred to as A6. This corresponds to a region in the roof of the tegmentum that is termed the **locus coeruleus.** The fluorescent technique has revealed that virtually all the cell bodies in this densely packed nucleus contain norepinephrine and give rise to fibers that traverse anteriorly in a pathway that Ungerstedt (1971) has referred to as the "dorsal tegmental bundle." Because of the possible confusion that can arise with later designations involving cholinergic fibers, this system will be referred to as the **dorsal noradrenergic bundle.**

The dorsal noradrenergic bundle projects anteriorly from the **locus coeruleus** before turning ventrally at about the level of the interpeduncular nucleus. The major portion of the bundle becomes incorporated into the **mammillary peduncle** and the **medial forebrain bundle.** Some of the fibers leave the bundle at the level of the interpeduncular nucleus to enter the **habenulo-interpeduncular tract** to terminate in the **lateral habenulae.** Somewhat more anteriorly, a smaller component of these fibers joins the **mammillothalamic tract** and terminates in the **anterior thalamic nucleus.** Lindvall and Björklund (1974) describe additional connections with the thalamus via fibers that enter the pretectal region (some of which cross in the posterior commissure) and with the ventrobasal aspects of the thalamus via fibers that travel adjacent to the medial lemniscus (see Fig. 11–1).

The remaining fibers of the dorsal noradrenergic bundle continue forward in the dorsomedial aspects of the medial forebrain bundle on its anterior course along the hypothalamus. Although some terminations are made within the hypothalamus, the bulk of the fibers is distributed to more anterior regions. A large component of the noradrenergic fibers leaves the region of the hypothalamus in a vertically oriented system to terminate in traditional limbic system structures. At the level of the anterior hypothalamus, fibers turn dorsally and project to the **anterior** and **reticular nuclei of the thalamus.** Some fibers terminate in the ventral aspect of the **bed nucleus of the stria terminalis,** but most of the fibers that traverse this region pass through the nucleus into the **stria terminalis** to eventually terminate in the **amygdala.** Slightly more anteriorly, fibers travel dorsally along the fornix columns; some of these fibers terminate in the caudal regions of the **septum,** but the major part of this system continues via the **fornix** to terminate in the **hippocampus.** Lindvall and Björklund (1974) report a smaller bundle that continues anteriorly from the rostral septum along the **intermediate olfactory tract** to terminate in the **anterior olfactory nucleus.**

Despite the numerous connections just described, a major portion of the original dorsal noradrenergic bundle remains at the level of the anterior septum. These fibers turn dorsally in the **septohypothalamic tract** and loop around the genu of the **corpus callosum** to join the **cingulum bundle.** As the cingulum travels posteriorly along the surface of the corpus callosum, fibers leave the bundle to terminate broadly throughout the cortex, and, eventually, the few remaining fibers loop around the splenium of the corpus callosum to enter the caudal region of the **hippocampus.**

The Ventral Noradrenergic Bundle. A second major system of norepinephrine-

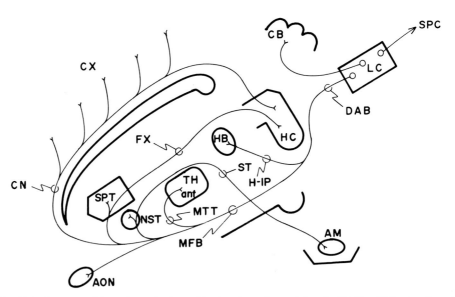

Fig. 11-1. Summary of the major projections of the dorsal noradrenergic bundle (DAB), which arises from the locus coeruleus (LC). The fibers make up portions of several major fiber tracts including the medial forebrain bundle (MFB), the mammillothalamic tract (MTT), the stria terminalis (ST), the fornix (FX), and the cingulum (CN). HB = habenula, ant = anterior regions of the thalamus (TH), NST = nucleus of the stria terminalis, AM = amygdala, SPT = septum, HC = hippocampus, AON = anterior olfactory nucleus, CX = cortex, CB = cerebellum, SPC = spinal cord.

109

HISTOCHEMICAL
MAPPING
OF THE
LIMBIC
SYSTEM

containing fibers arises from cell bodies that are located in several different regions of the brain stem. These regions were designated as areas A1, A2, A5, and A7 by Dahlström and Fuxe (1964).

Fibers from these regions converge near the base of the brain at the level of the interpeduncular nucleus to form what Ungerstedt (1971) referred to as the "ventral tegmental bundle." Again, to avoid possible confusion with later descriptions of the cholinergic systems, these fibers will be referred to as the **ventral noradrenergic bundle.** Before the fibers have converged, some fibers leave the scattered bundles to terminate in the **mesencephalic reticular formation** and the **central gray.** The remaining fibers form the ventrolateral aspect of the **medial forebrain bundle** near the posterior region of the hypothalamus. As the fibers course along the hypothalamus, numerous fibers leave the bundle to terminate in virtually all regions of the hypothalamus, but most notably in the **dorsomedial, periventricular, paraventricular, supraoptic,** and **arcuate nuclei** as well as in the **preoptic region.** Some fibers travel more laterally via the **ventral amyg-dalofugal pathway** or fibers of the **supraoptic decussation** to terminate in the **amygdala** and **pyriform cortex.** A smaller group of fibers travels along the internal capsule to terminate in the ventral regions of the **basal ganglia** and, rather specifically, in the **central nucleus of the amygdala.** The remaining fibers of the ventral noradrenergic bundle terminate in the **medial preoptic region** or the ventral aspects of the **bed nucleus of the stria terminalis** or join the diagonal band fibers to terminate in the **septum.** Apparently, none of the fibers terminates in the cortical regions or in the hippocampus, thus further differentiating the pattern of terminations from that of the dorsal noradrenergic bundle. These connections are summarized in Figure 11–2.

THE SEROTONERGIC SYSTEM

The cell bodies that contain serotonin are located primarily within the **dorsal raphe nucleus** of the central gray region, with some additional cells in the **medial raphe nucleus**

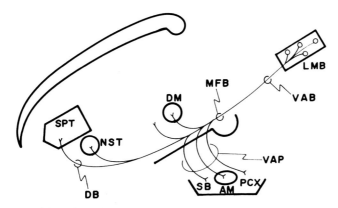

Fig. 11-2. Summary of the major projections of the ventral noradrenergic bundle (VAB), which originates in several different regions of the limbic midbrain (LMB). The fibers reach their points of termination via the medial forebrain bundle (MFB), the diagonal band (DB), and the ventral amygdalofugal pathway (VAP). DM = dorsomedial nucleus of the hypothalamus, PCX = pyriform cortex, AM = amygdala, SB = subiculum, NST = nucleus of the stria terminalis, SPT = septum.

and in the region of the **medial lemniscus** just posterior to the interpeduncular nucleus (see Fig. 11–3). These regions correspond to Dahlström and Fuxe's (1964) designations of B7, B8, and B9.

Ungerstedt (1971) has mapped out these systems in somewhat more detail. The fibers from the raphe region project anteriorly in the medial aspect of the tegmentum and then turn sharply ventrally at the level of the interpeduncular nucleus to join the **medial forebrain bundle.** From here, the projections seem to parallel those of the dorsal noradrenergic bundle to some extent, although the serotonergic system is somewhat less extensive. Two branches of fibers leave the medial forebrain bundle near the anterior regions of the hypothalamus to terminate in the **septum** and the **amygdala.** The remaining fibers loop around the genu of the **corpus callosum** to join the **cingulum** and terminate broadly throughout the cortex.

THE DOPAMINERGIC SYSTEM

The Nigrostriatal System

The cell bodies that contain dopamine are located primarily in the ventral tegmental region near the **substantia nigra** (see Fig. 11–4). The fibers that arise from cells located within the substantia nigra project anteriorly adjacent to the medial forebrain bundle. Although some of the fibers turn laterally to enter the **amygdala,** most of the fibers enter the **internal capsule** and distribute broadly within the **caudate-putamen.** The rather restricted source and projection of these fibers has led to its common designation as the "nigrostriatal system."

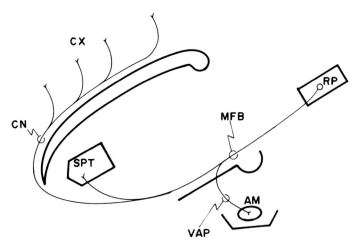

Fig. 11-3. Summary of the major projections of the serotonergic system that arises in the raphe nuclei (RP). The fibers travel in the medial forebrain bundle (MFB), the ventral amygdalofugal pathway (VAP), and the cingulum (CN) to terminate in the amygdala (AM), the septum (SPT), and the cortex (CX).

The Ventral Dopaminergic Bundle

111

HISTOCHEMICAL
MAPPING
OF THE
LIMBIC
SYSTEM

The cells that lie adjacent to the substantia nigra in the **ventral tegmental region** give rise to fibers that travel along the dorsal aspect of the **medial forebrain bundle.** At the level of the anterior hypothalamus, the fibers begin to disperse into rostral regions of the brain. One component of fibers turns laterally along the **ventral amygdalofugal pathway** to terminate in the **amygdala** and **pyriform cortex.** A second component merges with the **diagonal band** to terminate in the **lateral septum,** the **nucleus accumbens,** and, to a small extent, the **frontal cortex.** A third component continues anteriorly to terminate in the **olfactory tubercle.** There is a large component of fibers that joins the **septohypothalamic tract,** terminating in the **lateral septum, nucleus accumbens, anterior limbic cortex,** and **frontal cortex.**

THE ACETYLCHOLINE SYSTEMS

As previously mentioned, the rigid criteria for proving that a substance is a central nervous system neurotransmitter are virtually impossible to meet due to technical limitations. The most convincing evidence has been collected for acetylcholine, with numerous studies using a wide range of techniques. Ironically, acetylcholine is one of the more difficult compounds to study because it is extremely labile. Consequently, some of the methods that have been established for the investigation of cholinergic systems are indirect. Koelle (1954) developed a histochemical method that selectively stains the enzyme, acetylcholinesterase (AChE), which is chemically specific for the inactivation of acetylcholine. Because of the specificity of the enzyme, it is assumed that it would normally be

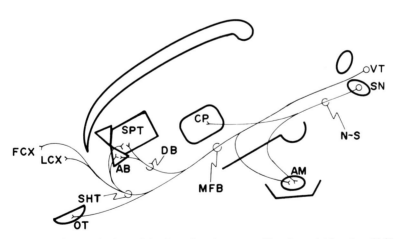

Fig. 11-4. Summary of the projections of the dopaminergic systems. The nigrostriatal system (N-S) projects from the substantia nigra (SN) to the caudate-putamen (CP) and amygdala (AM). Cells in the ventral tegmentum (VT) join the medial forebrain bundle (MFB) before branching out into the diagonal band (DB) and the septohypothalamic tract (SHT). SPT = septum, AB = nucleus accumbens, OT = olfactory tubercle, FCX = frontal cortex, LCX = lateral regions of the cortex.

present only in those systems that involve a cholinergic mechanism. Although there are some known exceptions to this restricted distribution, the method usually produces results that are highly correlated with known cholinergic systems in the periphery. Additionally, the method yields results that are comparable to those obtained with histochemical procedures based on choline acetylase, an enzyme involved in the synthesis of acetylcholine.

Most of the detailed mappings of central cholinergic pathways have been done by Shute and Lewis (e.g., Shute & Lewis, 1963, 1967; Lewis & Shute, 1967; Shute, 1973). The data they have collected are in basic agreement with electrophysiological, pharmacological, and bioassay data, which show a widespread distribution of cholinergic fibers within the brain. For the present purposes, the following summaries will be restricted to those cholinergic pathways that are directly involved with limbic system structures.

As in the case of the monoaminergic systems, the cells of origin of the cholinergic fiber systems are found in a fairly restricted portion of the brain stem. One cluster of cholinergic cells is located in the **cuneiform nucleus,** which is situated in the **dorsal tegmental region** just lateral to the central gray. These cells give rise to fibers that distribute widely within the optic tectum and the thalamus (especially midline regions). Shute and Lewis (1967) termed this system the ''dorsal tegmental pathway,'' which, for the present purposes, will be designated as the **dorsal cholinergic pathway.**

A second system arises from cells in the **substantia nigra** and adjacent regions of the **ventral tegmentum** and projects to the subthalamus, the thalamus, and a variety of limbic system structures including the cortex. This system will be designated as the **ventral cholinergic pathway.** These two major cholinergic pathways, schematized in Figure 11–5, may represent the thalamic and extrathalamic division of the reticular activating system that has been described using electrophysiological techniques (Domino, Dren, & Yamamoto, 1967).

As indicated in Figure 11–6, the cells of origin for the **ventral cholinergic pathway** arise from the **substantia nigra** and adjacent portions of the **ventral tegmental region** and project to a variety of basal forebrain structures. The fibers collect in the ventral tegmentum and project anteriorly along the lateral aspects of the hypothalamus. Several fiber components leave this system en route to establish synaptic connections with second-order cholinergic cells:

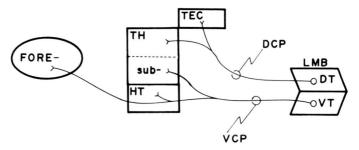

Fig. 11-5. Schematic summary of the cholinergic projections from the limbic midbrain regions (LMB). The dorsal cholinergic pathway (DCP) projects to the thalamus (TH) and tectum (TEC). The ventral cholinergic pathway (VCP) projects to the subthalamus (sub-), the thalamus (TH), and the hypothalamus (HT). DT = dorsal tegmentum, VT = ventral tegmentum.

113

HISTOCHEMICAL
MAPPING
OF THE
LIMBIC
SYSTEM

1. One component leaves the main body of fibers at the posterior border of the hypothalamus to terminate in the **supramammillary nuclei** and the **posterior hypothalamic nucleus.**

2. A second component leaves the main bundle somewhat more anteriorly and terminates on a cluster of cholinergic cells distributed throughout the **lateral hypothalamus, entopeduncular nucleus,** and **globus pallidus.**

3. A third component projects to a cluster of cholinergic cells that are distributed throughout the **lateral preoptic region** and the **bed nucleus** of the **stria terminalis.**

4. The remaining fibers continue anteriorly to terminate in the **islands of Calleja** and the **olfactory tubercle.**

In addition to these fibers that terminate on second-order cholinergic neurons, there are also a substantial number of fibers that terminate on noncholinergic neurons, particularly in the **paraventricular** and **supraoptic nuclei** of the hypothalamus.

Higher-Order Cholinergic Projections. Unlike the monoaminergic systems, which appear to project without interruption to rostral regions, the cholinergic fibers arising in the midbrain synapse with other cholinergic cells, which then project to more rostral regions. For the purposes of the present summary, the interconnections have been divided arbitrarily into cortical and subcortical projections.

The subcortical projections of the central cholinergic pathway arise primarily from second-order cells that are located in the **lateral preoptic region** and the ventral aspects of the **bed nucleus of the stria terminalis** (see Fig. 11–7). Fibers that arise from cells in these regions project to the **amygdala** via the **stria terminalis.** The largest system of fibers leaving the preoptic region project dorsally to terminate in the **nucleus of the diagonal band** and the **medial septal nucleus,** from which third-order cholinergic cells

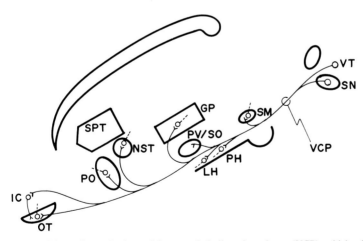

Fig. 11-6. Summary of the major projections of the ventral cholinergic pathway (VCP), which arises from the substantia nigra (SN) and adjacent regions of the ventral tegmentum (VT). SM = supramammillary nuclei, LH = lateral hypothalamus, PH = posterior hypothalamus, PV/SO = paraventricular/supraoptic region, GP = globus pallidus, NST = nucleus of the stria terminalis, PO = preoptic region, IC = islands of Calleja, OT = olfactory tubercle.

project posteriorly to terminate in the **hippocampus** and the **dentate gyrus.** In addition to these two major components of fibers, the lateral preoptic region also contributes fibers to the **nucleus** of the **lateral olfactory tract** and to the **nucleus accumbens,** the latter of which sends third-order fibers to the **olfactory tubercle.**

The **ventral cholinergic pathway** sends higher-order fibers to wide regions of the cortex (see Fig. 11–8). Fibers arising from cells in the **globus pallidus** project laterally through the external capsule to terminate in the **lateral cortex** just dorsal to the rhinal sulcus. The **amygdala** gives rise to fibers that also travel laterally but terminate in the **entorhinal cortex** and **pyriform cortex** just ventral to the rhinal sulcus. The most extensive cortical projection appears to arise from cells located in the **lateral preoptic region;** these fibers loop around the genu of the corpus callosum and project to the **cingulate cortex** and adjacent medial aspects of the cortical mantle. Some of these fibers travel more anteriorly to terminate in the **olfactory cortex,** but most of these anterior projections arise from cells located in the **olfactory tubercle** which project to both the **olfactory cortex** and the **olfactory bulbs** proper.

SUMMARY

The pathways that were described in this chapter were organized on the basis of their pharmacological characteristics. There are at least five major fiber systems that originate in the reticular formation and project rostrally into the limbic system:

1. The **ventral cholinergic pathway** projects from the cuneiform nucleus and adjacent regions to virtually all structures of the limbic system and to the neocortex. The system has been traced through a combination of histochemical, electrophysiological, pharmacological, and ablation procedures and appears to correspond to the **ascending reticular activating system.**

2. The **dorsal noradrenergic bundle** originates primarily in the locus coeruleus and projects along a pathway that is comparable to that of the ventral cholinergic pathway. There is considerable evidence that this system may be involved in a noradrenergic arousal system and, perhaps, in the mediation of reward processes.

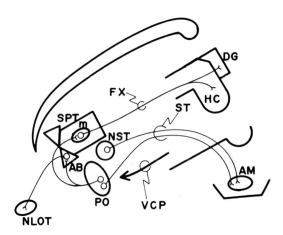

Fig. 11-7. Summary of the higher-order projections of the ventral cholinergic pathway (VCP) which terminate in subcortical regions. These fibers arise from cells in the preoptic nucleus (PO), the nucleus of the stria terminalis (NST), the nucleus accumbens (AB), and the medial septum (M). AM = amygdala, NLOT = nucleus of the lateral olfactory tract, HC = hippocampus, DG = dentate gyrus, FX = fornix, ST = stria terminalis.

115

HISTOCHEMICAL
MAPPING
OF THE
LIMBIC
SYSTEM

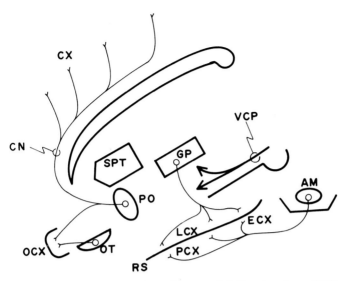

Fig. 11-8. Summary of the higher-order projections of the ventral cholinergic pathway (VCP) which terminate in cortical regions. The cell bodies are located in the amygdala (AM), globus pallidus (GP), preoptic nucleus (PO), and olfactory tubercle (OT). PCX = pyriform cortex, ECX = entorhinal cortex, RS = rhinal sulcus, LCX = lateral cortex, CN = cingulum, CX = cortex, OCX = olfactory cortex.

3. The **ventral noradrenergic bundle** originates in several different locations within the tegmentum and converges within the medial forebrain bundle before distributing projections to a variety of basal brain structures associated with the limbic system. This system has been implicated in the mediation of feeding behavior and possibly in the mediation of reward processes.

4. The **ventral dopaminergic pathway** arises from areas of the ventral tegmentum adjacent to the substantia nigra and projects to wide regions of the limbic system and neocortex. Recent data involving behavior in conjunction with pharmacological manipulations suggest that reward processes may be mediated by this dopaminergic system rather than by the noradrenergic systems.

5. The **serotonergic pathway** originates in the raphe system and projects to many of the same regions that receive projections from the diffuse noradrenergic, dopaminergic, and cholinergic systems. Data from several different sources suggest that this system may be involved in the mediation of sleep, punishment, and behavioral inhibition.

Comparisons of these pathways with the descriptions in previous chapters will reveal that, to a large extent, the same systems are being described. The pharmacologically defined pathways project via the traditional anatomically defined pathways, such as the habenulo-interpeduncular tract, the mammillary peduncle, the medial forebrain bundle, the fornix, and the cingulum. The organization based on the neurotransmitters provides an alternative view of these systems which may be either more convenient or more consistent with functional analyses than the structural approach. The next chapter will outline several different experimental approaches that will emphasize the alternative ways of conceptually organizing brain systems.

Some Fundamental Approaches to an Analysis of Limbic System Function

12

INTRODUCTION

In the preceding chapters it became apparent that the anatomical connections of the limbic system are so complex in their interactions that it is virtually impossible to view them as an integrated system. The original definition of the limbic system, as outlined by Broca in 1878, considered the limbic lobe to consist primarily of the septum, the cingulate cortex, and the hippocampal complex (refer to Fig. 1–1). Because of their seemingly close relationship with primary olfactory structures, the prevailing view at that time was that the limbic lobe was involved with higher-order olfactory processing. However, as anatomical methods became more precise, it was found that the olfactory bulbs did not contribute heavily to these structures (cf. Pribram & Kruger, 1954). These data, along with the classic paper by Papez (1937) suggesting a visceromotor function for these structures, led to a disuse of the term ''rhinencephalon.''

Papez' work, as well as a number of related experimental reports, stimulated much interest in the anatomy and function of the limbic system. The resulting discovery of new fiber pathways and behavioral data made it apparent that the initial boundaries of the limbic system were too restrictive. Virtually all of the shifting of boundaries has involved the addition of new structures; the only structure that has been dropped from the limbic system (and there is not general agreement on this) is the cingulate gyrus (see Chapter 10). Modern descriptions of the limbic system usually include the septohippocampal complex, the amygdala, several nuclei of the hypothalamus, parts of the thalamus, the frontal cortex, and several nuclei within the midbrain tegmentum (cf. Isaacson, 1974; Nauta, 1958, 1973). In light of the huge extent of the limbic areas, does it make sense to consider these complex structures and interconnections as a system?

117

The term "system" denotes a set of elements working together to mediate some type of function. Consider, for example, the meaning of the term in the case of the visual system. The fibers that interconnect the superior colliculus, the lateral geniculate, and the cortical projection regions constitute a system mediating a variety of electrophysiological and behavioral events, all of which are related to the process of vision. Similarly, the network of fibers interconnecting the precentral gyrus, the basal ganglia, and the cerebellum constitute a system that mediates reflexive, involuntary, and voluntary responses of both smooth and striated muscles. Here again, each individual element mediates somewhat different events, but in combination they are considered to perform a common function—that of muscular and glandular interaction with the environment. On a still more complex level, the hypothalamic circuits can be considered as systems that control various types of homeostatic processes. For example, experimental data indicate that hypothalamic nuclei are primarily involved in the regulation of such things as energy balance, water balance, electrolyte balance, and body temperature. Each of these is controlled by many factors, but it is conceptually useful to consider the hypothalamic circuits as being integral parts of a feeding system, a drinking system, a thermoregulatory system, etc.

In each instance outlined, the circuits described are considered to represent a system because each element is *essential* to some important aspect of the function. Surgical destruction of the lateral geniculate results in blindness, whereas destruction of the superior colliculus eliminates many visual reflexes. Similarly, damage in the precentral gyrus or the cerebellum will produce severe impairments in voluntary or reflexive motor responses. Destruction of the ventromedial nucleus of the hypothalamus will produce overeating and obesity, while damage in the lateral hypothalamus results in refusal to eat. (Additional examples and reviews may be found in secondary sources, such as Grossman, 1967, or Milner, 1970.)

If the limbic system can be realistically viewed as a system, then what essential function does it serve? As previously indicated, the limbic system is situated between the hypothalamic inputs associated with interoceptive information and the thalamocortical inputs associated with exteroceptive information (see Chapter 3). Furthermore, it is interconnected with structures that are involved with the motor output of the brain. However, the limbic system is not *essential* to any special sensory function, such as vision or olfaction, nor is it a necessary part of any homeostatic regulatory system; all of these functions can be retained following virtually any type of limbic system damage, and, additionally, primitive organisms lacking a limbic system can exhibit all of these basic functions.

There is general agreement that the major function of the limbic system is one of **modulation** of sensory, motor, and homeostatic systems (Isaacson, 1974; McCleary, 1966; Nauta, 1973). Typical of the data that support such a conclusion, it has been found that surgical destruction of the septum can (1) change food intake by altering the responsiveness to taste factors, internal cues, or reinforcement contingencies (cf. Beatty & Schwartzbaum, 1968; Hamilton, Capobianco, & Worsham, 1974): (2) change the responsiveness to environmental stimuli (cf. Brown & Remley, 1971); or (3) change certain types of motor responses (cf. McCleary, 1966). None of these effects represents a loss of the basic function but rather an impairment of some factor that controls the organism's response to that class of stimuli.

119

FUNDAMENTAL
APPROACHES TO
ANALYSIS OF
LIMBIC SYSTEM
FUNCTION

Nauta has suggested that the entire limbic system (including the frontal cortex, which he views as a sophisticated extension of the limbic system) functions as a sort of sounding board having the ability to preview alternative behaviors and evaluate the likely consequences. Given a certain situation, the limbic system may enable the organism to take into account the internal environment (e.g., depletion of energy stores) and the external environment (e.g., the presence of food) along with the events that would likely follow certain types of behaviors (e.g., potential attack by a predator). According to this view, the limbic system is integral in allowing the organism to cope with a complex and constantly changing environment. Clearly, this type of system superimposed on the basic sensory and regulatory systems has a great deal of survival value. For example, upon contact with food, a hungry organism is more likely to survive if it is able to take into account the current exigencies of the environment rather than eating immediately. It seems likely, then, that the limbic system is essential for the inhibition of otherwise prepotent responses.

The major advantages of classifying a set of anatomical structures as a system is to provide a conceptual framework that will aid in the organization of existing knowledge of brain function and to provide more systematic approaches to further research. A knowledge of the anatomical characteristics of a system is, perhaps, the single most important element in the design of research programs directed toward an understanding of function. Hopefully, the descriptions of limbic system circuitry in this text will provide students with a foundation for more fruitful research designs. The remaining sections of this chapter deal with fundamental approaches to the experimental analysis of the limbic system.

THE STRUCTURE–FUNCTION PROBLEM

Students of brain function have always hoped that the brain could somehow be parceled into individual units, each directly involved in the control of some specific type of behavior. If this were the case, then it would be a relatively simple matter to determine the functional correlates of brain structures in the same manner that physiologists have ascertained the function of the visceral organs. In some cases, this hope has been realized, as in the early demonstration of the function of the motor cortex (Fritsch & Hitzig, 1870), the somatosensory cortex, and the primary projection areas of the various sensory systems (e.g., Penfield & Rasmussen, 1950). For a time, it was thought that even more complicated behaviors, such as the regulation of feeding and drinking, were controlled by relatively circumscribed regions of the brain. For example, the classic studies of Hetherington and Ranson (1940) indicated that the ventromedial nucleus of the hypothalamus was largely responsible for the clinical obesity syndrome. These data, along with work by Anand and Brobeck (1951), suggested the existence of a lateral hypothalamic feeding center and a medial hypothalamic satiety center that controlled feeding behavior. With further research, however, it became apparent that this conceptualization of **centers** in the control of behavior was oversimplified. Robinson (1964) demonstrated that feeding could be elicited by electrical stimulation through electrodes located in virtually any area of the brain, especially limbic system sites. Numerous other studies have indicated that damage to limbic system structures, such as the septum and amygdala, can produce changes in feeding behavior. Thus, it became apparent that an understanding of the anatomical bases of these behaviors is much more complicated than was originally suspected. The notion of centers controlling certain behaviors has been replaced by the concept of **circuits** involving interactions among a number of different structures. Given the complex circuitry involved in various types of behavior, what are the best procedures for studying these relationships?

One of the oldest approaches to the investigation of the structure–function problem is the **ablation method.** The basic rationale is to compare the behavior of an intact organism with that of an organism that has incurred damage to some brain structure. If the brain-damaged organism is deficient in the performance of some task, then it is assumed that the structure was importantly involved in the normal regulation of that aspect of behavior.

This rationale is reasonably sound for the analysis of a system that is organized by centers for the control of simple behaviors. But as the anatomy and behavior become more complex, the limitations of the ablation method become apparent: The first problem encountered is that of anatomical specificity, which refers to the fact that virtually any type of brain damage will infringe upon overlapping circuits that serve different functions. The second problem is one of behavioral specificity, which refers to the fact that any particular behavioral task that is selected will involve more than one category of behavior. Let us examine these notions in more detail.

Anatomical Specificity

The major drawback of the ablation method is that it often interferes with a myriad of nuclei and their interconnections. This did not pose a serious problem to early investigators, who were simply trying to determine the general functional role of major subdivisions of the brain. As these descriptions became more precise, the need for greater anatomical precision was met with the development of the stereotaxic procedure (Horsely & Clark, 1908; Clark, 1939). Also, during recent years, a number of technical advances have been made which allow relatively discrete transection of fiber bundles rather than destroying nuclei (e.g., Albert, 1969; Sclafani & Grossman, 1969; Halasz & Pupp, 1965; Hamilton, Worsham, & Capobianco, 1973; Hamilton & Timmons, 1976). None of these techniques is sufficiently precise to avoid damage to overlapping circuits, but all can be used in combination with other procedures as a powerful approach to studying the behavioral correlates of specific nuclei and fiber tracts. The basic rationale of this approach is to systematically assess the effects of damage in several different regions of a circuit. Each locus of damage will involve the destruction of adjacent systems, but the sites can be selected so that the only feature in common is the single system that is being investigated.

A knowledge of the origins, projection pathways, and fields of termination of the various pathways can suggest several alternative ways of dissecting a system, some of which may be more efficient than others. For example, a change in behavior following extensive septal damage could be based upon any of several different circuits interconnecting the septum with other structures. If, for example, the effect is based on the connections between the medial septum and the hippocampus, then animals with discrete medial septal lesions or fornix transections should show similar effects on the behavioral mea-

121

FUNDAMENTAL
APPROACHES TO
ANALYSIS OF
LIMBIC SYSTEM
FUNCTION

sure. Alternatively, the behavioral change might be based upon the interconnections of the lateral septum with the hypothalamus, in which case animals with damage restricted to the lateral septal nuclei would share some of the changes that occur following undercutting of the septum. Once the directionality of the system has been determined, more detailed manipulations can be performed to subdivide this aspect of the system.

A similar approach can be used to investigate a particular fiber system. For example, if the transection of the stria terminalis just above the bed nucleus produces a specific behavioral change, the possibility exists that the change could be due to inadvertent damage to adjacent structures, such as the septum, thalamus, or stria medullaris. These alternatives can be ruled out by interrupting the same system at different points (e.g., by producing a lesion in the bed nucleus of the stria terminalis, by transecting the bundle of fibers as it descends near the hippocampus, or by producing lesions in the points of origin within the amygdaloid complex).

A point of logic regarding the ablation method is so simple that it deserves mention only because it is so frequently overlooked. The rhetoric is awkward, but one does not study the effects of a lesion—one studies the ability of the remaining brain tissue to control behavior. There are subtle problems of interpreting the normal functional significance of the tissue that is missing, and these problems are compounded by the fact that the remaining tissue does not remain static. Degenerative changes influence the anatomical and pharmacological integrity of distant locations, adjacent tissue may be stimulated to establish new fiber connections, and other portions of the brain may compensate for deficits through alternative behaviors. The time course of these changes may range from several hours to several weeks or months. Accordingly, caution must be exercised in assigning specific functions to specific circuitry unless the data are corroborated by studies of detailed anatomical changes, pharmacological assays, and appropriate controls for postoperative recovery time (see Schoenfeld & Hamilton, 1977).

Behavioral Specificity

Most behavioral tasks selected for assessing the effects of central nervous system manipulation (e.g., ablation) involve many different aspects of behavior. For example, suppose an animal must learn to avoid electric shock by jumping over a barrier each time a light is presented. If a brain-damaged animal is deficient in the acquisition of this task, it could be postulated that the region that was destroyed is normally involved in forming associations between environmental stimuli. However, before such a conclusion can be reached, it is necessary to control for alternate explanations, such as the possibility that the organism has a visual deficit making it more difficult to see the warning signal, a motor deficit that makes it difficult to negotiate the barrier, or an elevated threshold for pain which makes the electric shock less aversive. Even if these relatively simple alternatives can be ruled out, the behavioral deficit could be attributed to an altered emotional response to the aversive situation or to a deficit in the ability to initiate responses of any kind.

Although it is possible to control for most of the alternatives cited, conclusions must still be tempered to reflect the possibility that organisms may utilize different cues or strategies in learning the same task. For example, a complex maze task may be learned on the basis of proprioceptive cues (e.g., the series of left and right turns), intramaze cues (e.g., odors or markings on the floor and walls of the maze), or extramaze cues (e.g., spatial relationship to overhead lights, doors, or sources of noise). Although these may appear to be minor points, there is some indication that there are differences within a species so that female rats tend to use extramaze cues, whereas male rats rely more heavily on intramaze cues (cf., White & McGee, personal communication). Clearly, differences such as these would have to be taken into account in any attempts to correlate maze-learning ability with neuroanatomical structures.

As indicated, it is often difficult to make conclusive statements about behavioral specificity since, even in apparently simple situations, the behavior of organisms is based on complex reactions to the environment. The only way to parcel out a specific type of behavior is to investigate a number of different types of behavioral tasks which all appear to have one aspect in common. A particularly relevant example of this approach is McCleary's (1966) review of the role of the septohippocampal complex in behavioral inhibition. McCleary reviews a variety of experimental situations that all required the inhibition of responding. In some cases, the tests involved electrical shock in passive avoidance, punishment, one-way avoidance, or two-way avoidance. In other cases, the tests involved nonreinforcement in instrumental or operant situations using various types of cues to signal the presence or absence of reinforcement. The results of any one of these experiments could be attributed to changes in the response to painful shock, to various types of sensory information, to food deprivation, or to the reinforcing properties of food. As McCleary points out, some of these changes in responsiveness occur following septal lesions, but considering the range of tests, the only explanation that can account for all of the observed behavioral changes is the notion that the animals with damage to the septohippocampal system have an impaired ability to inhibit punished or nonrewarded responses. This deficit in behavioral inhibition following septal lesions represents a common factor across all the experiments, thereby assuming the status of an **intervening variable.** Although the approach outlined here is tedious, it is probably the only successful way to analyze the complex behavioral changes that accompany neural damage. The intervening variables established by this approach are useful, because they can be used to predict behavioral changes in other situations that require the same class of behaviors.

Combining Anatomical and Behavioral Specificity

There are two extreme alternatives that can be used in correlating behavior and anatomy. One approach is to produce damage to a specific structure and determine the effects of this manipulation on all possible types of behavior. The other is to test animals on one type of behavior and determine the effects of damage to all possible sites within the brain. Each method is inefficient, and most investigators adopt a heuristic approach and investigate a select number of similar behaviors in association with different types of damage to related neural structures. With this method, it is frequently possible by inference to fill in the gaps along either the behavioral or anatomical dimension.

In some cases, a preliminary knowledge of the possible function of a particular circuit can allow an investigator to use a particularly powerful approach called the **double-dissociation design.** An example of this is an experiment performed by McCleary (1961) based on earlier findings by Kaada (1951). The Kaada experiments had demonstrated that stimulation of the cingulate gyrus facilitated spinal motor reflexes, whereas

123

FUNDAMENTAL
APPROACHES TO
ANALYSIS OF
LIMBIC SYSTEM
FUNCTION

stimulation of the septal region inhibited spinal reflexes. McCleary reasoned that the surgical removal of these regions would produce opposite effects on motor responses. In one case, the behavioral task required that the animal perform an active motor response in order to avoid electrical shock; in the other, the animal could avoid shock only by passively refraining from responding. In this experiment, normal cats, cats with cingulate lesions, and cats with septal lesions were tested on both response measures. The cats with cingulate damage were normal or slightly better than normal in the passive avoidance task but were impaired in the active avoidance task. Conversely, the cats with septal lesions were normal or slightly better than normal in the performance of the active response but were impaired in the ability to passively avoid shock. If McCleary's experiment had involved only one of the lesion groups, the resulting deficit could be attributed to nonspecific effects due to surgery, altered response to shock, or the possibility that one task is more sensitive than the other in detecting behavioral deficits. Separate experiments would have been needed to investigate each of these alternatives. However, the opposing patterns of deficits obtained when both manipulations are used in the double-dissociation design allow one to rule out these possibilities in a very efficient manner.

PHARMACOLOGICAL APPROACHES

In the preceding chapter, several pharmacological systems were described that have their origins in the midbrain and project rostrally into limbic structures. The existence of these circuits has obviously prompted speculation that different pharmacologically based systems may have different functional significance. Thus, any technique that can selectively influence a particular pharmacological system may serve as an important tool for correlating behavioral function with a particular transmitter system. Although it is likely that a single transmitter system may have an anatomical organization that allows it to participate in more than one function, it is still possible, on the basis of much empirical evidence, to attribute specific functions to each of the major transmitter systems:

Cholinergic fibers have been implicated in behavioral inhibition (cf. Carlton, 1963), behavioral arousal (cf. Shute & Lewis, 1967), and the regulation of water intake (cf. Grossman, 1964).

Noradrenergic fiber systems appear to be involved in behavioral arousal (cf. Weiss & Laties, 1962), reward mechanisms (cf. Stein, 1968), and the regulation of feeding behavior (cf. Grossman, 1964).

Dopaminergic fibers regulate motor functions of the extrapyramidal system (cf. Krauthamer, 1975; McLennan, 1970) and possibly reward mechanisms (cf. Crow, 1972).

Serotonergic fibers have been implicated in behavioral inhibition (cf. Carlton & Advokat, 1975) and in the regulation of certain aspects of sleep (cf. Jouvet, 1972).

Each of the neurotransmitter systems is chemically specific in terms of the synthesis and inactivation of the transmitter substance. Furthermore, the pharmacological compounds that influence the neurotransmitter are also different in each case (cf. Cooper, Bloom, & Roth, 1970; Goodman & Gilman, 1965; Myers, 1972). Irrespective of the system that is being investigated, the drugs can be grouped according to the type of effect they have on the transmitter system. For the present purposes, a brief rationale will be given for the use of several different categories of pharmacologically active compounds.

Drugs That Mimic or Enhance Neurotransmitter Action

Because of the chemical specificity of the transmitter systems, certain drugs can be administered to mimic the action of the neurotransmitter. Unlike electrical stimulation, chemical stimulation only influences a particular subpopulation of neurons based on the chemical specificity of the receptor sites. Although this specificity can be attained with systemic administration of the drugs, even further specificity can be achieved if the effect is restricted to a small anatomical region by injecting the drug directly into a discrete region of the brain. Behavioral changes that accompany the administration of these compounds may be the result of activation of the neurons that normally control this type of behavior. Yet, caution must be exercised in the interpretation of these experiments, because the application of the drug will not necessarily induce a pattern of neural activity that is essential for the normal functioning of the circuits involved.

The logic of these arguments is somewhat more compelling in the case of manipulations that do not directly stimulate the postsynaptic receptors but rather make the system more effective during its normal activity. This effect can be achieved through several mechanisms, including an increase in the production and storage of the transmitter, a decrease in the effectiveness of the inactivation mechanism (either enzymatic degradation or re-uptake), or the replacement of the neurotransmitter stores with a false transmitter that is more effective than the endogenous transmitter. Although all of these procedures seem, logically, to involve an exaggerated form of normal function, there are still problems of interpretation and dose levels are critical. In some systems, a slight increase in the amount of transmitter substance may have no effect in terms of the functional result. Moderate increases may, in fact, produce the desired enhancement of function. However, if the dosage is too high, the excess transmitter substance may actually induce a blockade of function rather than a facilitation.

Drugs That Block or Deplete the Neurotransmitter

Chemical compounds that block the effects of a neurotransmitter released during normal activity produce effects that are similar to, but more selective than, that which occurs following surgical destruction. The advantage of this approach is that these compounds only block the function of certain chemically specific neurons. Furthermore, the compounds usually do not induce distant changes such as those accompanying the degenerative phenomena that follow surgical damage. As in the case of stimulating compounds, more selective effects can be obtained if the compound is injected directly into a brain region that is believed to contain the appropriate type of neurons.

Other classes of pharmacologically active compounds act by depleting a system of its transmitter stores rather than by blocking the effects of transmitter release. Essentially, the same types of results can be expected since the system would no longer be capable of functioning in its normal capacity. A particularly interesting compound that can be included in this category is 6-hydroxy-dopamine (6-OH-DA). This drug appears to rather specifically attack and destroy the synaptic terminals that utilize either dopamine or norepinephrine as the neurotransmitter (cf. Mandel, Mack, & Goridis, 1975).

The use of blocking agents rather than agents that mimic the neurotransmitter may represent a somewhat more powerful technique for determining the function of a transmitter system. With the administration of a blocking agent, it is logical to assume the **absence** of normal function in the affected system, whereas the application of a mimicking agent does not necessarily imply the exaggerated **presence** of normal function.

Specificity of Action

Every pharmacologically active compound has multiple effects. Although the major effect of a compound may be to block Transmitter A, it may additionally block Transmitter B or stimulate the receptors for Transmitter C. Depending on the experimental bias of the investigator, one of these effects will be considered the main effect and the other two will be termed "side effects." Since the behavioral effects of a compound are likely to be no more selective than the pharmacological effects, the problem of specificity is again present. To some extent, these problems can be circumvented by using several different compounds that share some common property (e.g., the blockade of Transmitter B) but which have differing "side effects." Using this approach, any behavioral commonality among the compounds may be attributable to some similarity in the pharmacological actions of the drugs. These arguments, of course, apply irrespective of the route of administration of the compounds.

Another successful approach is to use different drugs in combination or in succession. For example, if it appears that a particular behavior may be under the control of a system utilizing Transmitter A, then a compound that is known to block Transmitter A could be administered. If a second drug manipulation still produces the behavior that is being investigated, then it is likely that the second drug is producing its effects via its actions on another transmitter system.

Still another approach is to take advantage of the anatomical distribution of a particular neurotransmitter system. For example, the cells of origin for the dorsal noradrenergic bundle are located in the locus coeruleus, while those of the ventral noradrenergic bundle are located in the more ventral regions of the tegmentum. Thus, surgical destruction of the locus coeruleus should produce some, but not all, of the behavioral changes that follow the systemic administration of drugs that block noradrenergic activity. Drug-induced behavioral changes that are not paralleled by locus coeruleus damage are probably due to the drug's action on the ventral noradrenergic system.

In all of these approaches, the power of the techniques is limited by the specificity of the behavior being studied. Thus, the same cautions and rationale discussed in regard to behavioral specificity are equally applicable here.

PHYLOGENETIC APPROACHES

The brains of organisms at different points on the phylogenetic scale differ greatly with respect to the size and structural characteristics of the major subdivisions. As described in Chapter 3, the spinal cord and midbrain regions are relatively constant across fish, amphibia, reptiles, birds, and mammals, whereas the limbic system and neocortical mantle show progressive development along the phylogenetic scale. MacLean (1952,

125

FUNDAMENTAL
APPROACHES TO
ANALYSIS OF
LIMBIC SYSTEM
FUNCTION

1970) has formalized these observations and incorporated them with evolutionary theory to develop the concept of the **triune brain.** The phylogenetic implications are clear in MacLean's designations of the **reptilian brain** (brain stem), the **paleomammalian brain** (diencephalon and limbic system), and the **neommalian brain** (neocortex). To the extent that there are consistent differences in behavior associated with a particular level of brain development, the comparative behavioral approach could be a powerful approach for determining at least the general functions of certain brain regions.

One of the major drawbacks to this approach is that the behavior of different organisms is closely attuned to a particular environmental niche, irrespective of similarities or differences in brain structure. Not only are there certain innate behavior patterns, but there are also differences in certain behavioral propensities involved in learned behavior. For example, given a choice, rats will use tactile or olfactory stimuli to perform a task, whereas birds rely more on visual cues. Moreover, the motor capabilities and response topographies differ greatly as a function of species. In light of all these differences, can the comparative study of behavior add anything to our knowledge of structure–function relationships?

One of the most successful approaches to this problem is Bitterman's (cf. 1965) analysis of the ability to perform successive reversals. In these experiments, the organism was trained to choose between two stimuli, one associated with reward and the other with nonreward. After learning this discrimination, the reward conditions were reversed so that the animal had to shift to the opposite stimulus to obtain reward. In these experiments, the rate of learning, the type of apparatus, and the nature of the reward differed greatly, because the organisms that were tested included fish, birds, rats, monkeys, humans, and even elephants. Bitterman designed these experiments so that the nature of the response, the type of reward, and even the absolute rate of learning were unimportant. The critical aspect of the experiment was the *relative* rate of learning successive reversals. Fish and lower organisms showed no improvement with successive reversals—each discrimination required about the same number of trials to learn. Some birds, however, showed a gradual improvement, eventually responding to the shifted reward conditions within a few trials. Monkeys, rats, and humans showed great improvement in this ability, eventually responding to the shifted reward conditions after a single trial.

Bitterman's results are important because they point out progressive differences in a complex form of learning that parallel the relative positions on the phylogenetic scale. It seems likely that these differences may also parallel those which occurred over the course of evolution and strongly suggest that the rapid expansion of the limbic system and neocortex may be the anatomical substrate for this behavioral development.

ONTOGENETIC APPROACHES

The ontogenetic development of the brain parallels the apparent course of phylogenetic development in that the rostral regions reach functional maturity at progressively later stages (see Fig. 3–2). This process, called **encephalization,** continues over a fairly long period of time after birth in some mammals, allowing the opportunity to assess the behavioral capabilities of the organism at different ages and to correlate structural de-

127

FUNDAMENTAL
APPROACHES TO
ANALYSIS OF
LIMBIC SYSTEM
FUNCTION

velopment with the appearance of certain types of behaviors. During the past decade, this approach has been extremely useful in providing insights into the functional aspects of certain parts of the limbic system.

The most straightforward approach in this area is simply to measure a particular behavior at various ages to determine when the behavioral capability reaches mature levels. Studies of this type have shown a fairly consistent pattern of sensory and motor development across a wide range of species (cf. Gottlieb, 1971). The fact that sensory and motor systems may not be fully developed at the time of behavioral testing creates some problems, but the careful selection of tasks can ensure that the lack of maturity of these systems will not bias the results.

Campbell and his associates (Campbell, Lytle, & Fibiger, 1969; Mabry & Campbell, 1974) have performed a series of experiments that exemplify the power of combining different methodologies and provide data concerning the functional and pharmacological characteristics of the limbic system. The rationale of the behavioral aspects of the experiments was that locomotor activity can be increased either by an increase in excitation (e.g., via amphetamine administration) or by blocking inhibition (e.g., by atropine or scopolamine administration). These effects had already been verified in adult rats (cf. Carlton, 1963). Campbell *et al.* (1969) found that amphetamine increased the activity of rat pups at all ages tested, 10 days being the earliest age. By contrast, cholinergic blockade was ineffective until the rats were 18–21 days of age. A similar time course for development has also been shown for the behavioral responsiveness to cholinergic blockade on passive avoidance responding (Feigley, 1974) and for the habituation of exploratory responding (cf. Williams, Hamilton & Carlton, 1975; Feigley, Parsons, Hamilton, & Spear, 1972). More recently, data have shown that manipulations involving the serotonergic system become effective as early as 10–12 days of age (cf. Mabry & Campbell, 1974) and may influence simpler types of inhibitory behaviors such as the habituation of the reflexive startle response (e.g., Carlton & Advokat, 1974; Williams *et al.*, 1975).

Another type of combined approach involving the developing brain is the investigation of the effects of brain damage produced at various ages. In many cases, the behavioral deficits that accompany specific lesions are much more severe if the damage is produced in adulthood than if it is produced during early development; this is especially true if the damage occurs before the behavior in question is fully developed (cf. Harlow, Blomquist, Thompson, Schiltz, & Harlow, 1968; Isaacson, Nonneman, & Schmaltz, 1968; White, 1972). Although there are some exceptions to this type of results (e.g., Schoenfeld, Hamilton, & Gandelman, 1974), the developing brain appears to be able to compensate for the missing tissue much better than the fully matured brain. Further investigations of this type, especially in conjunction with anatomical studies of neuronal sprouting, may be an unusually fruitful area for future research.

CONCLUSIONS

The intersection of several different approaches with the study of behavioral development have contributed greatly to our understanding of limbic system organization:

(1) The ablation method has demonstrated the functional significance of many limbic system pathways and has opened the possibility that alternative pathways are available in the developing brain; (2) histological techniques involving stains for degenerating fibers and histofluorescent techniques have demonstrated that the limbic system is interconnected with the brain stem via several pharmacologically distinct sets of fibers; (3) both the development of certain behaviors and the interaction of specific drugs with these behaviors indicate that these fiber systems develop at different rates and in some cases do not reach functional maturity for several weeks after birth; (4) chemical assays have corroborated these findings by demonstrating that several of the enzyme systems involved in the synthesis or inactivation of certain neurotransmitters follow the same time course; and (5) studies of the neuronal substructure have shown that certain limbic structures, such as the hippocampus and frontal cortex, show relatively late dendritic development and myelinization, the time course of which also parallels that of behavioral development.

Taken together, these data suggest different developmental timetables and functions for the major transmitter systems that arise in the midbrain and project to rostral limbic sites. The progressively later development of these ascending systems is probably determined by the physical growth and myelinization of these neurons as well as by the development of metabolic systems associated with the transmitter substances. Finally, since the sequence of the ontogenetic development seems to parallel that of phylogenetic development, the data from these studies have important implications for an understanding of the evolutionary history of behavioral capabilities.

Appendix: A Bibliographic Guide to Further Study of the Limbic System

The purpose of this text, as indicated in the preface, is to provide an overview of the essential anatomical characteristics of the limbic system and related structures. In an effort to avoid unnecessary detail and maintain a reasonable level of readability, the number of references in the text was kept to a minimum. However, it is recognized that some readers will require additional information on a particular topic for the purpose of research or the preparation of seminar papers. This bibliographic guide is designed to facilitate these types of literature searches. Although the list of references that follows is in no sense exhaustive, it should lead the reader to virtually all major publications in the field. In addition to the first section of the bibliography, which is organized according to chapter headings, there is a second section, which contains a list of atlases of the rat brain, a list of major textbooks in neuroanatomy, and a list of technical journals that are likely to contain recent references.

PART I: REFERENCES PERTAINING TO INDIVIDUAL CHAPTERS

Chapter 1: A Brief History of the Study of Neuroanatomy (Pp. 1–6)

The history of anatomy and anatomists can be found in a variety of historical and bibliographical sources. Most of these are to be found under the general heading of medical history rather than under more specific neuroanatomical headings. The following references represent a sampling of some of the more relevant and interesting treatments of the subject:

Boring, E.G. *A History of Experimental Psychology.* New York, Appleton-Century-Crofts, 1950.

Haymaker, W., & Schiller, F. (Eds.) *The Founders of Neurology.* Springfield, Thomas, 1970.

Lind, L.R. (translator) *The Epitome of Andreas Vesalius.* Cambridge, M.I.T. Press, 1969

Riese, W., & Hoff, E.C. A history of the doctrine of cerebral localization. II. Methods and main results. *J. Hist. Med. Allied Sci., 6:*439–470, 1951.

Rosner, B.S. Recovery of function and localization of function in historical perspective. In Stein, D.G., Rosen, J.J., & Butters, N. (Eds.): *Plasticity and Recovery of Function in the Central Nervous System.* New York, Academic Press, 1974.

Poynter, F.N.L. (Ed.) *The History and Philosophy of Knowledge of the Brain and Its Functions.* Springfield, Thomas, 1958.

Singer, C.J. *A Short History of Anatomy from the Greeks to Harvey.* New York, Dover, 1957.

Walker, A.E. Stimulation and ablation: their role in the history of cerebral physiology. *J. Neurophysiol. 20:*435–449, 1957.

Young, R.M. *Mind, Brain and Adaptation in the Nineteenth Century. Cerebral Localization and Its Biological Context from Gall to Ferrier.* Oxford, Clarendon Press, 1970.

The classic theoretical papers that ultimately led to the notion of the limbic system are as follows:

Broca, P. Anatomie comparée des circonvolutions cérébrales. Le grand lobe limbique et la scissure limbique dans la série des mammifères. *Rev. Anthropol., 1:*385–498, 1878.

Clark, G. The use of the Horsely-Clark instrument on the rat. *Science, 90:*92, 1939.

Herrick, C.J. The functions of the olfactory parts of the cortex. *Proc. Nat. Acad. Sci, 19:*7–14, 1933.

Hetherington, A.W., & Ranson, S.W. Hypothalamic lesions and adiposity in the rat. *Anat. Rec., 78:*149, 1940.

Horsely, V., & Clark, R.H. The structure and functions of the cerebellum examined by a new method. *Brain, 31:*45–124, 1908.

Klüver, H., & Bucy, P.C. An analysis of certain effects of bilateral temporal lobectomy in the rhesus monkey with special reference to "psychic blindness." *J. Psychol., 5:*33–54, 1938.

Kölliker, A. *Handbuch der Gewebelehre des Menschen.* Leipzig, Wilhelm Engelman, 1870.

Lashley, K.S. In search of the engram. *Proc. Soc. Exp. Biol. Med. 4:*454–482, 1950.

Papez, J.W. A proposed mechanism of emotion. *Arch. Neurol. Psychiat., 38:*725–743, 1937.

Pribram, K.H., & Kruger, L. Functions of the "olfactory brain." *Ann. N.Y. Acad. Sci., 58:*109–138, 1954.

Major textbooks of neuroanatomy (mostly based on human anatomy) and a list of rat brain atlases may be found in the second portion of this bibliography (see pp. 143 and 144.) Those specifically referenced in this chapter include:

Crosby, E.C., Humphrey, T., & Lauer, E.W. *Correlative Anatomy of the Nervous System.* New York, Macmillan, 1962.

Ranson, S.W., & Clark, S.L. *The Anatomy of the Nervous System.* Philadelphia, Saunders, 1959.

Truex, R.C. *Human Neuroanatomy.* Baltimore, Williams & Wilkins, 1969.

Chapter 2: Neuroanatomical Procedures and Terminology (Pp. 7–23)

The most comprehensive and thorough treatment of modern techniques in neuroanatomy can be found in the excellent collection edited by Nauta and Ebbesson (1970). The relevant sections of this text should be read as a first step in gaining a more thorough appreciation of the problems and interpretation of anatomical procedures. Because of its particular importance to this topic, the reference for the text and the table of contents are listed below:

Nauta, W.J.H., & Ebbesson, S.O.E. (Eds.) *Contemporary Research Methods in Neuroanatomy.* New York, Springer-Verlag, 1970.

1. The rapid Golgi method. Indian summer or renaissance? (Scheibel, M.E., & Scheibel, A.B.)
2. The Golgi method. A tool for comparative structural analyses. (Valverde, F.)
3. The Golgi-Cox technique. (Ramón-Moliner, E.)

4. The fixation of central nervous tissue and the analysis of electron micrographs of the neuropil, with special reference to the cerebral cortex. (Peters, A.)
5. Light- and electron-microscopical studies of normal and degenerating axons. (Guillery, R.W.)
6. Selective silver-impregnation of degenerating axoplasm. (Heimer, L.)
7. The selective silver-impregnation of degenerating axons and their synaptic endings in nonmammalian species. (Ebbesson, S.O.E.)
8. Bridging the gap between light and electron microscopy in the experimental tracing of fiber connections. (Heimer, L.)
9. Neuronal changes central to the site of axon transection. A method for the identification of retrograde changes in perikarya, dendrites, and axons by silver-impregnation. (Grant, G.)
10. Electron microscopy of Golgi preparations for the study of neuronal relations. (Blackstad, T.W.)
11. Anterograde and retrograde transneuronal degeneration in the central and peripheral nervous system. (Cowan, W.M.)
12. Autoradiographic methods and principles for study of the nervous system with thymidine-H^3. (Sidman, R.L.)
13. Flourescence microscopy in neuroanatomy. (Fuxe, K., Hökfelt, T., Jonsson, G., & Ungerstedt, U.)
14. Methods for the counting of neurons. (Konigsmark, B.W.)

Primary sources for various anatomical and histological procedures (refer also to references relating to Chapter 11) include:

Bielschowski, M. Die Silberimprägnation der Neurofibrillen. J. Psychol. Neurol. (Lpz.), 4:169–188, 1904.
Blackstad, T.W. Electron microscopy of experimental axon degeneration in photochemically modified Golgi preparations: a procedure for precise mapping of nervous connections. *Brain Res., 95:*191–210, 1975.
Brazier, M.A.B. *The Electrical Activity of the Nervous System.* New York, Macmillan, 1961.
Clark, G. The use of the Horsely-Clark instrument on the rat. *Science, 90:*92, 1939.
Cowan, W.M., Gottlieb, D.I., Hendrickson, A., Price, J.L., & Woolsey, T.A. The autoradiographic demonstration of axonal connections in the central nervous system. *Brain Res., 37:*21–51, 1972.
de Olmos, J.S. The amygdaloid projection field in the rat as studied with the cupric-silver method. In Eleftheriou, B.E. (Ed.): *The Neurobiology of the Amygdala,* New York, Plenum Press, 1972.
Falck, B. Observations on the possibilities of the cellular localization of monoamines by a flourescent method. *Acta Physiol. Scand., 56:*1–25, 1962 (Suppl. 197).
Falck, B., Hillarp, N.A., Theme, G., & Torp, A. Flourescence of catecholamines and related compounds condensed with formaldehyde. *J. Histochem. Cytochem., 10:*348–354, 1962.
Fink, R.P., & Heimer, L. Two methods for selective silver impregnation of degenerating axons and their synaptic endings in the central nervous system. *Brain Res., 4:*369–374, 1967.
Fuxe, K., Hökfelt, T., Jonsson, G., & Ungerstedt, U. In Nauta, W.J.H., and Ebbesson, S.O.E. (Eds.): *Contemporary Research Methods in Neuroanatomy.* New York, Springer-Verlag, 1970.
Klüver, H., & Barrera, E.A. A method for the combined study of cells and fibers in the nervous system. *J. Neuropath. Exp. Neurol., 12:*400–403, 1953.
Lavail, J.H. The retrograde transport method. *Fed. Proc., 34:*1618–1624, 1975.
Lewis, P.R., Shute, C.C.D., & Silver, A. Confirmation from choline acetylase analyses of a massive cholinergic innervation to the rat hippocampus. *J. Physiol. Lond., 191:*215–224, 1967.
Lynch, G., Gall, C., Mensah, P., & Cotman, C.W. Horseradish peroxidase histochemistry: a new method for tracing efferent projections in the central nervous system. *Brain Res., 65:*373–380, 1974.
Nauta, W.J.H., & Ebbesson, S.O.E. (Eds.) Contemporary Research Methods in Neuroanatomy. New York, Springer-Verlag, 1970. For a listing of chapter titles, see the previous section.
Nauta, W.J.H. Silver impregnation of degenerating axons. In Windle, W.F. (Ed.): *New Research Techniques of Neuroanatomy,* Springfield, Thomas, 1957.
Nauta, W.J.H., & Gygax, P.A. Silver impregnation of degenerating axons in the central nervous system: a modified technique. *Stain Technol., 29:*91–93, 1954.
Nitsch, C., & Bak, I.J. Moss fiber endings of Ammon's horn, demonstrated with the freeze etching technic. *Verh. Anat. Ges., 68:*319–323, 1974 (Ger.).
Powell, E.W., & Schnurr, R. Silver impregnation of degenerating axons; comparisons of postoperative intervals, fixatives, and staining methods. *Stain Technol., 47:*95–100, 1972.
Raisman, G. Neuronal plasticity in the septal nuclei of the adult rat. *Brain Res., 14:*25–48, 1969.
Sherlock, D.A., & Raisman, G. A comparison of anterograde and retrograde axonal transport of horseradish peroxidase in the connections of the mammillary nuclei in the rat. *Brain Res., 85:*321–324, 1975.

Shute, C.C.D. Cholinergic pathways of the brain. In Laitinen, L.V., & Livingston, K.E. *Surgical Approaches to Psychiatry,* Baltimore, University Park Press, 1972.

Shute, C.C.D., & Lewis, P.R. Cholinesterase-containing systems of the brain of the rat. *Nature (Lond.), 199*:1160–1164, 1963.

Ungerstedt, U. Stereotaxic mapping of the monoamine pathways in the rat brain. *Acta Physiol. Scand., 82*:1–48, 1971 (Suppl. 367).

van Harreveld, A., & Fifkova, E. Swelling of dendritic spines of the fascia dentata after stimulation of the perforant fibers as a mechanism of post-tetanic potentiation. *Exp. Neurol., 49*:736–749, 1975.

Some useful secondary sources for histological and anatomical research techniques include the following:

Drury, R.A.B., & Wallington, E.A. *Carlton's Histological Technique.* New York, Oxford University Press, 1967.

Myers, R.D. (Ed.) *Methods in Psychobiology: Vols. 1 and 2.* New York, Academic Press, 1971 and 1972.

Ruch, T.C., Patton, H.D., Woodbury, J.W., & Towe, A.L. *Neurophysiology.* Philadelphia, Saunders, 1961.

Singh, D., & Avery, D.D. *Physiological Techniques in Behavioral Research.* Monterey, Cal., Brooks-Cole, 1975.

Webster, W.G. *Principles of Research Methodology in Physiological Psychology.* New York, Harper & Row, 1975.

Wolf, G. Elementary histology for neuropsychologists. In Myers, R.D. (Ed.): *Methods in Psychobiology, Vol. 1,* New York, Academic Press, 1971.

Chapter 3: The Limbic System Defined (Pp. 25–32)

In many respects, this is the most difficult chapter to supplement with references because there are no clear boundaries. The concept of the limbic system has evolved in the context of anatomical connections, developmental and evolutionary observations, as well as physiological and behavioral functions. The references cited below include sources from a wide range of areas and should provide an industrious reader with several hundred additional references.

General Overviews and Terminology:

Andy, O.J., & Stephan, H. The septum in the human brain. *J. Comp. Neurol., 133*:383–410, 1968.

Broca, P. Anatomie comparée des circonvolutions cérébrales. Le grand lobe limbique et la scissure limbique dans la série des mammifères. *Rev. Anthropol, 1*:385–498, 1878.

Elliot Smith, G. The morphology of the limbic lobes, corpus callosum, septum pellucidum and fornix: a preliminary communication. *J. Anat. Physiol., 30*:157–167, 1896.

Elliot Smith, G. The term "archipallium"—a disclaimer. *Anat. Anz., 35*:429, 1910.

Foville, A.L. *Traité complet de l'anatomie de la physiologie et de la pathologie du système nerveux cérébro-spinal.* Paris, Masson, 1844.

Livingston, K.E., & Escobar, A. Anatomical bias of the limbic system concept. A proposed reorientation. *Arch. Neurol., 24*:17–21, 1971.

MacLean, P.D. Some psychiatric implications of physiological studies of the fronto-temporal portion of the limbic system (visceral brain). *Electroencephalog. Clin. Neurophysiol., 4*:407–418, 1952.

MacLean, P.D. The triune brain, emotion and scientific bias. In Schmidt, F.O. (Ed.): *The Neurosciences Second Study Program,* New York, Rockefeller University Press, pp. 336–348, 1970.

Moore, J.C. Behavior bias and the limbic system. *Am. J. Occup. Ther., 30*:11–19, 1976.

Nauta, W.J.H. Hippocampal projections and related neural pathways to the midbrain in the cat. *Brain, 81*:319–340, 1958.

Nauta, W.J.H. Connections of the frontal lobe with the limbic system. In Laitinen, L.V., & Livingston, K.E. (Eds.): *Surgical Approaches in Psychiatry,* Baltimore, University Park Press, 1973.

Owen, R. *Anatomy of Vertebrates.* London, Longmans & Green, 1868.

Papez, J.W. A proposed mechanism of emotion. *Arch. Neurol. Psychiat., 38*:725–744, 1937.

Powell, E.W., & Hines, G. The limbic system: an interface. *Behav. Biol., 12*:149–164, 1974.

Powell, T.P.S. Sensory convergence in the cerebral cortex. In Laitinen, L.V., & Livingston, K.E. (Eds.): *Surgical Approaches in Psychiatry,* Baltimore, University Park Press, 1973.

Raisman, G. An evaluation of the basic pattern of connections between the limbic system and the hypothalamus. *Am. J. Anat., 129*:197–201, 1970.

Riggs, A. Nomica Generica. *Science, 190*:612, 1975.

Riss, W., Halpern, M., & Scalia, F. Anatomical aspects of the evolution of the limbic and olfactory systems and their potential significance for behavior. *Ann. N.Y. Acad. Sci., 159*:1096–1111, 1969.

Schwalbe, G. *Lehrbuch der Neurologie.* Erlangen, Germany, Besold, 1881.

Teuber, H.L. Unity and diversity of frontal lobe functions. *Acta Neurobiol. Exp. (Warsz.), 32*:615–656, 1972.

Tilney, F. The hippocampus and its relations to the corpus callosum. *Bull. Neurol. Inst. N.Y., 7*:1–77, 1938.

Turner, W. The convolutions of the brain: a study in comparative anatomy. *J. Anat. Physiol., 25*:105–154, 1890.

Wald, G. Biochemical evolution. In Barron, E.S.G. (Ed.): *Modern Trends in Physiology and Biochemistry,* New York, Academic Press, p. 339, 1952.

White, L.E., Jr. A morphological concept of the limbic lobe. *Int. Rev. Neurobiol., 13*:1–34, 1970.

Ontogenetic and Phyologenetic Development:

The references listed below consist primarily of technical papers devoted to specific topics relating to the morphological and biochemical aspects of development. (The reader should cross-reference with the preceding section and with references relating to Chapters 2 and 11. The section following will deal with behavioral references.):

Altman, J. & Das, G.D. Autoradiographic and histological evidence of postnatal hippocampal neurogenesis in rats. *J. Comp. Neurol., 124*:319–336, 1965.

Altman, J., & Das, G.D. Autoradiographic and histological studies of postnatal neurogenesis. I. A longitudinal investigation of the kinetics, migration and transformation of cells incorporating tritiated thymidine in neonate rats, with special reference to postnatal neurogenesis in some brain regions. *J. Comp. Neurol., 126*:337–389, 1966.

Appel, S.H. Neuronal recognition and synaptogenesis. *Exp. Neurol., 48*:52–74, 1975.

Bayer, S.A., & Altman, J. Hippocampal development in the rat: cytogenesis and morphogenesis examined with autoradiography and low-level x-irradiation. *J. Comp. Neurol., 158*:55–79, 1974.

Bliss, T.V., Chung, S.H., & Stirling, R.V. Proceedings: structural and functional development of the mossy fiber system in the hippocampus of the postnatal rat. *J. Physiol. (Lond.), 239*:92P–94P, 1974.

Crain, B., Cotman, C., Taylor, D., & Lynch, G. A quantitative electron microscopic study of synaptogenesis in the dentate gyrus of the rat. *Brain Res., 63*:195–204, 1973.

Das, G.D. Experimental studies on the postnatal development of the brain. I. Cytogenesis and morphogenesis of the accessory fascia dentata following hippocampal lesions. *Brain Res., 28*:263–282, 1971.

Diamond, M.C., Johnson, R.E., & Ingham, C.A. Morphological changes in the young, adult, and aging rat cerebral cortex, hippocampus, and diencephalon. *Behav. Biol., 14*:163–174, 1975.

Dzidzishvili, N.N., & Kvirkvelia, L.R. Electrophysiological signs of hippocampal development ontogenesis. *Prog. Brain Res., 22*:414–426, 1968.

Gottlieb, D.I., & Cowan, W.M. Evidence for a temporal factor in the occupation of available synaptic sites during the development of the dentate gyrus. *Brain Res., 41*:452–456, 1972.

Gregory, E. Comparison of postnatal CNS development between male and female rats. *Stain Technol., 50*:152–156, 1975.

Humphrey, T. Correlations between the development of the hippocampal formation and the differentiation of the olfactory bulbs. *Ala. J. Med. Sci., 3*:235–269, 1966.

König, N., Roch, G., & Marty, R. The onset of synaptogenesis in rat temporal cortex. *Anat. Embryol. (Berl.), 148*:73–87, 1975.

Kretschman, H.J., & Wingert, F. On the quantitative development of hippocampal formation in the albino rat. *J. Hirnforsch., 10*:471–486, 1968 (Ger).

Krug, H., & Wenk, H. Changes in the feulgen hydrolysis curve during postnatal growth in the hippocampus of the rat. *Acta Histochem. (Jena), 45*:305–321, 1973 (Ger).

Lauder, J.M., & Bloom, F.E. Ontogeny of monoamine neurons in the locus coeruleus, raphe nuclei and substantia nigra of the rat. II. Synaptogenesis. *J. Comp. Neurol., 163*:251–264, 1975.

Matthews, D.A., Nadler, J.V., Lynch, G.S., & Cotman, C.W. Development of cholinergic innervation in the hippocampal formation of the rat. I. Histochemical demonstration of acetylcholinesterase activity. *Devel. Biol., 36*:130–141, 1974.

Mellgren, S.I. Distribution of acetylcholinesterase in the hippocampal region of the rat during postnatal development. *Z. Zellforsch. Mikrosk. Anat., 141*:375–400, 1973.

Minkwitz, H.G., & Holz, L. The ontogenetic development of pyramidal neurons in the hippocampus (CA1) of the rat. *J. Hirnforsch., 16*:37–54, 1975.

Meyer, U., Ritter, J., & Wenk, H. Chemodifferentiation of the hippocampal formation in the postnatal development of albino rats. I. Oxydoreductases. *J. Hirnforsch., 13*:235–253, 1971 (Ger).

Nadler, J.G., Matthews, D.A., Cotman, C.W., & Lynch, G.S. Development of cholinergic innervation in the hippocampal formation of the rat. II. Quantitative changes in choline acetyltransferase and acetylcholinesterase activities. *Devel. Biol., 36*:142–154, 1974.

Ritter, J., Meyer, U., & Wenk, H. Chemodifferentiation of the hippocampus formation in the postnatal development of albino rats. II. Transmitter enzymes. *J. Hirnforsch., 13*:254–278, 1971 (Ger).

Sarnat, H.B., & Netsky, M.G. *Evolution of the Nervous System.* New York, Oxford University Press, 1974.

Schlessinger, A.R., Cowan, W.M., & Gottlieb, D.I. An autoradiographic study of the time of origin and the pattern of granule cell migration in the dentate gyrus of the rat. *J. Comp. Neurol., 159*:149–175, 1975.

Sorimachi, M., Miyamoto, K., & Kataoka, K. Postnatal development of choline uptake by cholinergic terminals in rat brain. *Brain Res., 79*:343–346, 1974.

Vaughan, D.W., & Peters, A. Neuroglial cells in the cerebral cortex of rats from young adulthood to old age: an electron microscope study. *J. Neurocytol., 3*:405–429, 1974.

Westrum, L.E. Electron microscopy of synaptic structures in olfactory cortex of early postnatal rats. *J. Neurocytol., 4*:713–732, 1975.

Westrum, L.E. Axonal patterns in olfactory cortex after olfactory bulb removal in newborn rats. *Exp. Neurol., 47*:442–447, 1975.

Functional Correlates of the Limbic System:

The study of the functions of the limbic system comprises a major portion of a broad area of research known as physiological psychology. The books and technical articles cited below include secondary sources that contain many additional references and a selection of technical articles that are especially consistent with the author's biases:

Altman, J., Bruner, R.L., & Bayer, S.A. The hippocampus and behavioral maturation. *Behav. Biol., 8*:557–596, 1973.

Boakes, R.A., & Halliday, M.S. (Eds.) *Inhibition and Learning.* New York, Academic Press, 1972.

Campbell, B.A., Lytle, L.D., & Fibiger, H.C. Ontogeny of adrenergic arousal and cholinergic inhibitory mechanisms in the rat. *Science, 166*:635–637, 1969.

Eleftheriou, B.E. (Ed.) *The Neurobiology of the Amygdala.* New York, Plenum Press, 1975.

Gregory, E.H., & Pfaff, D.W. Development of olfactory-guided behavior in infant rats. *Physiol. Behav., 6*:573–576, 1971.

Grossman, S.P. *A Textbook of Physiological Psychology.* New York, Wiley, 1967.

Hockman, C.H. (Ed.) *Limbic System Mechanisms and Autonomic Functions.* Springfield, Thomas, 1967.

Isaacson, R.L. (Ed.) *Basic Readings in Neuropsychology.* New York, Harper & Row, 1964.

Isaacson, R.L. *The Limbic System.* New York, Plenum Press, 1974.

Isaacson, R.L., & Pribram, K.H. (Eds.) *The Hippocampus:* Vol. 1, *Structure and Development,* Vol. 2, *Physiology and Behavior.* New York, Plenum Press, 1975.

Kimble, D.P. Hippocampus and internal inhibition. *Psychol. Bull., 70:*285–295, 1968.

Mabry, P.D., & Campbell, B.A. Ontogeny of serotonergic inhibition of behavioral arousal in the rat. *J. Comp. Physiol. Psychol., 86*:193–201, 1974.

Milner, P.M. *Physiological Psychology.* New York, Holt, Rinehart & Winston, 1970.

Stellar, E., & Sprague, J.M. (Eds.) *Progress in Physiological Psychology,* Vols. 1 & 2. New York, Academic Press, 1966 & 1968.

Tapp, J.T. (Ed.) *Reinforcement and Behavior.* New York, Academic Press, 1969.

Thompson, R.F. *Introduction to Physiological Psychology.* New York, Harper & Row, 1975.

Tobach, E., Aronson, L.R., & Shaw, E. (Eds.) *The Biopsychology of Development.* New York, Academic Press, 1971.

Williams, J.M., Hamilton, L.W., & Carlton, P.L. Pharmacological and anatomical dissociation of two types of habituation. *J. Comp. Physiol. Psychol., 87*:724–732, 1974.

Williams, J.M., Hamilton,, I.W., & Carlton, P.L. An ontogentic analysis of two classes of habituation. *J. Comp. Physiol. Psychol., 89:*733–737, 1975.

Zeman, W., & Innes, J.R.M. *Craigie's Neuroanatomy of the Rat.* New York, Academic Press, 1963.

Chapter 4: General Topography of the Limbic System (Pp. 33–52)

Brodal, A. The hippocampus and the sense of smell. A Review. *Brain, 70:*179–222, 1947.

MacLean, P.D. Some psychiatric implications of physiological studies of the fronto-temporal portion of the limbic system (visceral brain). *Electroencephalog. Clin. Neurophysiol., 4:* 407–418, 1952.

Chapter 5: The Fornix System and Related Hippocampal Connections (Pp. 53–62)

The hippocampal complex and closely related structures, such as the septum and the entorhinal cortex, represent the most intensively studied portion of the limbic system. As indicated in the references relating to Chapter 3, the hippocampus has served as the anatomical substrate for a disproportionately large share of the developmental and behavioral studies (the reader should cross-reference). In addition, some of the most imaginative and sophisticated approaches to the study of the nervous system have used the hippocampal complex as a testing ground (cross-reference with Chapters 2 and 12). The reader is also referred to a thorough collection of papers edited by Isaacson and Pribram (1975, see Chapter 3). The technical articles selected for inclusion in the list below are those that deal primarily with the delineation of hippocampal connections:

Blackstad, T.W. Commissural connections of the hippocampal region of the rat, with special reference to their mode of termination. *J. Comp. Neurol., 105:*417–537, 1956.

Cruce, J.A. An autoradiographic study of the projections of the mammillothalamic tract in the rat. *Brain Res., 85:*211–219, 1975.

Deadwyler, S.A., West, J.R., Cotman, C.W., & Lynch, G.S. A neurophysiological analysis of commissural projections to the dentate gyrus of the rat. *J. Neurophysiol., 38:*167–184, 1975.

deFrance, J.F., Shimono, T., & Kitai, S.T. Anatomical distribution of the hippocampal fibers afferent to the lateral septal nucleus. *Brain Res., 34:*176–180, 1971.

Goldowitz, D., White, W.F., Steward, O., Lynch, G.S., & Cotman, C.W. Anatomical evidence for a projection from the entorhinal cortex to the contralateral dentate gyrus of the rat. *Exp. Neurol., 47:*433–441, 1975.

Gottlieb, D.I., & Cowan, W.M. Autoradiographic studies of the commissural and ipsilateral association connections of the hippocampus and dentate gyrus. I. The commissural connections. *J. Comp. Neurol., 149:*393–422, 1973.

Guillery, R.W. Degeneration of the post-commissural fornix and the mammillary peduncle of the rat. *J. Anat. Lond., 90:*350–370, 1956.

Hjorth-Simonsen, A. Hippocampal efferents to the ipsilateral entorhinal area: an experimental study in the rat. *J. Comp. Neurol., 142:*417–438, 1971.

Hjorth-Simonsen, A. Some intrinsic connections of the hippocampus in the rat: an experimental analysis. *J. Comp. Neurol., 147:*145–162, 1973.

Hjorth-Simonsen, A., & Jeune, B. Origin and termination of the hippocampal perforant path in the rat studied by silver impregnation. *J. Comp. Neurol., 144:*215–232, 1972.

Lindvall, O. Mesencephalic dopaminergic afferents to the lateral septal nucleus of the rat. *Brain Res., 87:*89–95, 1975.

Lorente de Nó, R. Studies on the structure of the cerebral cortex. II. Continuation of the study of the ammonic system. *J. Psychol. Neurol. (Lpz.), 46:*113–117, 1934.

Lynch, G.S., Stanfield, B., Parks, T., & Cotman, C.W. Evidence for selective post-lesion axonal growth in the dentate gyrus of the rat. *Brain Res., 69:*1–11, 1974.

Meibach, R.C., & Siegel, A. The origin of fornix fibers which project to the mammillary bodies in the rat: a horseradish peroxidase study. *Brain Res., 88:*508–512, 1975.

Mosko, S., Lynch, G.S., & Cotman, C.W. The distribution of septal projections to the hippocampus of the rat. *J. Comp. Neurol., 152*:163–174, 1973.

Nauta, W.J.H. An experimental study of the fornix system in the rat. *J. Comp. Neurol., 104*:247–270, 1956.

Nauta, W.J.H. Hippocampal projections and related neural pathways to the midbrain in the cat. *Brain, 81*:319–340, 1958.

Nauta, W.J.H., & Haymaker, W. Hypothalamic nuclei and fiber connections. In Haymaker, W., Anderson, E., & Nauta, W.J.H. (Eds.): *The Hypothalamus*, Springfield, Thomas, 1969.

Raisman, G. The connexions of the septum. *Brain, 89:*317–348, 1966.

Raisman, G., Cowan, W.M., & Powell, T.P.S. The extrinsic afferent, commissural, and association fibers of the hippocampus. *Brain, 88*:963–996, 1965.

Raisman, G., Cowan, W.M., & Powell, T.P.S. An experimental analysis of the efferent projection of the hippocampus. *Brain, 89*:83–108, 1966.

Segal, M. Hippocampal unit responses to perforant path stimulation. *Exp. Neurol., 35*:541–546, 1972.

Segal, M., & Landis, S. Afferents to the hippocampus of the rat studied with the method of retrograde transport of horseradish peroxidase. *Brain Res., 78*:1–15, 1974.

Segal, M., & Landis, S. Afferents to the septal area of the rat studied with the method of retrograde axonal transport of horseradish peroxidase. *Brain Res., 82*:263–268, 1974.

Siegal, A., Edinger, H., & Ogami, S. The topographical organization of the hippocampal projection to the septal area: a comparative neuroanatomical analysis in the gerbil, rat, rabbit and cat. *J. Comp. Neurol., 157*:359–377, 1974.

van Harreveld, A., & Fifkova, E. Swelling of dendritic spines of the fascia dentata after stimulation of the perforant fibers as a mechanism of post-tetanic potentiation. *Exp. Neurol., 49*:736–749, 1975.

Zimmer, J., & Hjorth-Simonsen, A. Crossed pathways from the entorhinal area to the fascia dentata. II. Provokable in rats. *J. Comp. Neurol., 161*:71–101, 1975.

Zimmer, J. Extended commissural and ipsilateral projections in postnatally deentorhinated hippocampus and fascia dentata demonstrated in rats by silver impregnation. *Brain Res., 64*:293–311, 1973.

Zimmer, J. Changes in the Timm sulfide silver staining pattern of the rat hippocampus and fascia dentata following early postnatal deafferentation. *Brain Res., 64*:313–326, 1973.

Chapter 6: Connections of the Stria Medullaris and Habenulae (Pp. 63–72)

The habenular nuclei per se have been the object of only a few direct studies. In addition to the references cited below, the reader should cross-reference with articles describing the circuitry of the septum and the limbic midbrain:

Akagi, K. & Powell, E.W. Differential projections of habenular nuclei. *J. Comp. Neurol., 132*:263–274, 1968.

Cragg, B.G. The connections of the habenula in the rabbit. *Exp. Neurol., 3:*388–409, 1961.

Gurdjian, E.S. The diencephalon of the albino rat. *J. Comp. Neurol., 43*:1–114, 1927.

Leranth, C.S., Brownstein, M., Aborsky, L., Aranyi, Z.S., & Palkovits, M. Morphological and biochemical changes in the rat interpeduncular nucleus following transection of the habenulo-interpedunculo tract. *Stain Technol., 50*:124–128, 1975.

Marburg, O. The structure and fiber connections of the human habenula. *J. Comp. Neurol., 80*:211–233, 1944.

Massopust, L.C., Jr., & Thompson, R. A new interpedunculo-diencephalic pathway in rats and cats. *J. Comp. Neurol., 118*:97–106, 1962.

Nauta, W.J.H., & Haymaker, W. Hypothalamic nuclei and fiber connections. In Haymaker, W., Anderson, E., & Nauta, W.J.H. (Eds.): *The Hypothalamus*, Springfield, Thomas, 1969.

Chapter 7: The Stria Terminalis, the Ventral Amygdaloid Pathways, and Related Amygdaloid Connections (Pp. 73–78)

The amygdala has been difficult to study anatomically owing to its complex substructure and somewhat inaccessible location. Despite these differences, numerous behavioral studies have been conducted, anticipating the later definition of many of the amygdaloid connections. The reader is referred to secondary sources listed in Part II of this bibliography for behavioral references. The most comprehensive treatment of the anatomy of the amygdala can be found in B.E. Eleftheriou's (1972) collection of papers entitled *The Neurobiology of the Amygdala* (New York, Plenum Press, 1972). Additional sources include:

Brodal, A. The amygdaloid nucleus in rat. *J. Comp. Neurol., 87*:1–16, 1947.

Cowan, W.M., Raisman, G., & Powell, T.P.S. The connexions of the amygdala. *J. Neurol. Neurosurg. & Psychiat., 28*:137, 1965.

de Olmos, J.S. The amygdaloid projection field in the rat as studied with the cupric-silver method. In Eleftherious, B.E. (Ed.): *The Neurobiology of the Amygdala,* New York, Plenum Press, 1972.

de Olmos, J.S., & Ingram, W.R. The projection field of the stria terminalis in the rat brain. An experimental study. *J. Comp. Neurol., 146*:303–334, 1972.

Druga, R. Neocortical projections to the amygdala. (An experimental study with the Nauta method.) *J. Hirnforsch., 11*:467–476, 1969.

Girgis, M. The amygdala and the sense of smell. *Acta Anat. (Basel), 72*:502–519, 1969.

Gurdjian, E.S. The diencephalon of the albino rat. *J. Comp. Neurol., 43*:1–114, 1927.

Hall, E. Some aspects of the structural organization of the amygdala. In Eleftheriou, B.E. (Ed.): *The Neurobiology of the Amygdala,* New York, Plenum Press, 1972.

Heimer, L., & Nauta, W.J.H. The hypothalamic distribution of the stria terminalis in the rat. *BrainRes., 13*:284–297, 1969.

Johnston, J.B. Further contribution to the study of the evolution of the forebrain. *J. Comp. Neurol., 35*:337–481, 1923.

Krettek, J.E., & Price, J.L. Projections from the amygdala to perirhinal and entorhinal cortices and the subiculum. *Brain Res., 71*:150–154, 1974.

Leonard, C.M., & Scott, J.W. Origin and distribution of the amygdalofugal pathways in the rat: an experimental neuroanatomical study. *J. Comp. Neurol., 141*:313–330, 1971.

Loo, Y.T. The forebrain of the opossum, *Didelphius virginiana,* Part I. Gross anatomy. *J. Comp. Neurol., 51*:13–64, 1930.

Nauta, W.J.H., & Haymaker, W. Hypothalamic nuclei and fiber connections. In Haymaker, W., Anderson, E., & Nauta, W.J.H. (Eds.): *The Hypothalamus.* Springfield, Thomas, 1969.

Nitecka, L. Comparative aspects of the localization of acetylcholinesterase activity in the amygdaloid body. *Folia Morphol. (Warsz.), 34*:167–185, 1975.

Parent, A. Comparative histochemical study of the amygdaloid complex. *J. Hirnforsch., 13*:89–96, 1971.

Rae, A.S. Histology of the zone of contact between amygdala and hippocampus. *Confin. Neurol., 31*:330–333, 1969.

Chapter 8: The Medial Forebrain Bundle and Related Hypothalamic Connections (Pp. 79–85)

The interconnections of the hypothalamus and the medial forebrain bundle with other regions of the brain are so extensive that it is necessary to cross-reference virtually every chapter in this text. Special notice should be given to the references cited for Chapters 5, 7, and 11. The most comprehensive treatment of the hypothalamus and related fiber paths can be found in:

Haymaker, W., Anderson, E., & Nauta, W.J.H. (Eds.) *The Hypothalamus.* Springfield, Thomas, 1969. (See especially, Chapter 4 by Nauta and Haymaker.)

A selection of other useful sources includes:

Clark, W.E.L. *The Hypothalamus.* London, Oliver & Boyd, 1938.

Gurdjian, E.S. The diencephalon of the albino rat. *J. Comp. Neurol., 43*:1–114, 1927.

Heimer, L., & Nauta, W.J.H. The hypothalamic distribution of the stria terminalis in the rat. *Brain Res., 13*:284–297, 1969.

Knook, H.L. *The Fiber Connections of the Forebrain.* Assen, van Gorcum & Co. N. V., 1965.

Lammers, H.J., & Lohman, A.H. Structure and fiber connections of the hypothalamus in mammals. *Prog. Brain Res., 41*:61–78, 1974.

Leonard, C.W., & Scott, J.W. Origin and distribution of the amygdalofugal pathways in the rat: an experimental study. *J. Comp. Neurol.*, *141:*313–330, 1971.

Loo, Y.T. The forebrain of the opossum, *Didelphius virginiana,* Part I. Gross anatomy. *J. Comp. Neurol.*, *51:*13–64, 1930.

Chapter 9: The Lateral Olfactory Tract, the Anterior Commissure, and Other Olfactory Connections (Pp. 87–93)

Since the olfactory system is closely related to the habenula, amygdala, and hypothalamus, the reader is advised to cross-reference Chapters 6, 7, and 8. Although a wealth of information is available concerning the characteristics of olfactory reception and the olfactory control of behavior, the present list of references includes primarily those directly related to anatomical descriptions:

Allison, A.C. The structure of the olfactory bulb and its relations to the olfactory pathways in the rabbit and the cat. *J. Comp. Neurol.*, *98:*309–353, 1953.

Brodal, A. The hippocampus and the sense of smell. *Brain, 70:*179–222, 1947.

Brodal, A. The origin of fibers of the anterior commissure in the rat. Experimental studies. *J. Comp. Neurol.*, *88:*157–205, 1948.

DeVries, H., & Stuiver, M. The absolute sensitivity of the human sense of smell. In Rosenblith, W.A. (Ed.): *Sensory Communication,* New York, Wiley, 1959, pp. 159–167.

Druga, R. Projection area of the olfactory bulb in the rat. *Folia Morphol. (Praha), 21:*328–329, 1973.

Druga, R. The projection field of the prepyriform cortex (an experimental study using Nauta's method). *Folia Morphol. (Praha), 20:*169–171, 1972.

Ferrer, N.G. Efferent projections of the anterior olfactory nucleus. *J. Comp. Neurol.*, *137:*309–320, 1969.

Gurdjian, E.S. Olfactory connections in the albino rat, with special reference to the stria medullaris and the anterior commissure. *J. Comp. Neurol.*, *38:*127–163, 1925.

Heimer, L. The olfactory connections of the diencephalon in the rat. An experimental light- and electron-microscopic study with special emphasis on the problem of terminal degeneration. *Brain Behav. Evol.*, *6:*484–523, 1972.

Land, J.L., Eager, R.P., & Shepherd, G.M. Olfactory nerve projections to the olfactory bulb in rabbit: demonstration by means of a simplified ammoniacal siver degeneration method. *Brain Res., 23:*250–254, 1970.

Lohman, A.H., & Mentink, G.M. The lateral olfactory tract, the anterior commissure and the cells of the olfactory bulb. *Brain Res., 12:*396–413, 1969.

Milner, P.M. *Physiological Psychology.* New York, Holt, Rinehart & Winston, 1970.

Minckler, J. *Introduction to Neuroscience.* St. Louis, Mosby, 1972.

Nicoll, R.A. Recurrent excitatory pathways of anterior commissure and mitral cell axons in the olfactory bulb. *Brain Res., 19:*491–493, 1970.

Powell, T.P.S., Cowan, W.M., & Raisman, G. The central olfactory connexions. *J. Anat., 99:*791–813, 1965.

Price, J.L. The origin of the centrifugal fibers to the olfactory bulb. *Brain Res., 14:*542–545, 1969.

Price, J.L., & Powell, T.P. An electron-microscopic study of the termination of the afferent fibres to the olfactory bulb from the cerebral hemisphere. *J. Cell Sci., 7:*157–187, 1970.

Price, J.L., & Powell, T.P. An experimental study of the origin and course of the centrifugal fibres to the olfactory bulb in the rat. *J. Anat. 107:*215–237, 1970.

Price, J.L., & Powell, T.P. The afferent connexions of the nucleus of the horizontal limb of the diagonal band. *J. Anat., 107:*239–256, 1970.

Price, J.L., & Sprich, W.W. Observations on the lateral olfactory tract of the rat. *J. Comp. Neurol., 162:*321–336, 1975.

Raisman, G. An experimental study of the projection of the amygdala to the accessory olfactory bulb and its relationship to the concept of a dual olfactory system. *Exp. Brain Res., 14:*395–408, 1972.

Scalia, F., & Winans, S.S. The differential projections of the olfactory bulb and accessory olfactory bulb in mammals. *J. Comp. Neurol., 161:*31–55, 1975.

Scott, J.W., & Chafin, B.R. Origin of olfactory projections to lateral hypothalamus and nuclei gemini of the rat. *Brain Res., 88:*64–68, 1975.

Shepherd, G.M. Synaptic organization of the mammalian olfactory bulb. *Physiol. Rev., 52:*864–917, 1972.

Sinclair, J.G. Reflections on the role of receptor systems for taste and smell. *Int. Rev. Neurobiol., 14:*159–171, 1971.

Thamke, B., Schulz, E. & Schönheit, B. Neurohistological studies on the olfactory bulb of the adult white laboratory rat (Rattus norvegicus, forma alba). *J. Hirnforsch., 14:*435–449, 1973.

Tucker, G.F., Jr., Alonso, W.A., Cowan, M., Tucker, J.A., & Druck, N. The anterior commissure revisited. *Ann. Otol. Rhinol. Laryngol., 82:*625–636, 1973.

Chapter 10: Cortical Extensions of the Limbic System (Pp. 95–103)

Several aspects of the cortex are closely interrelated to specific aspects of the limbic system, and the reader is advised to cross-reference with other chapters, especially Chapters 5, 7, 9, and 11. Although there are many articles dealing with descriptions of the anatomical characteristics of the cortex per se, the references cited below have been selected because they emphasize the relationship to the limbic system:

Abbie, A.A. The relations of the fascia dentata, hippocampus and neocortex and the nature of the subiculum. *J. Comp. Neurol., 68:*307–323, 1938.

Clark, W.E. Le Gros. An experimental study of the thalamic connections in the rat. *Trans. Roy. Soc. Lond., 222B:*1–28, 1932.

Clark, W.E. Le Gros, & Boggon, R.H. On the connections of the anterior nucleus of the thalamus. *J. Anat. (Lond.), 67:*215–226, 1933.

Domesick, V.B. Projections of the cingulate cortex in the rat. *Brain Res., 12:*296–320, 1969.

Domesick, V.B. The fasciculus cinguli in the rat. *Brain Res., 20:*19–32, 1970.

Hjorth-Simonsen, A. Hippocampal efferents to the ipsilateral entorhinal area: an experimental study in the rat. *J. Comp. Neurol., 142:*417–438, 1971.

Krieg, W.J.S. Connections of the cerebral cortex. I. The albino rat. A. Topography of cortical area. *J. Comp. Neurol., 81:*221–247, 1946.

Krieg, W.J.S. Connections of the cerebral cortex. I. The albino rat. C. Extrinsic connections. *J. Comp. Neurol., 86:*267–294, 1947.

Leonard, C.M. The prefrontal cortex of the rat. I. Cortical projection of the mediodorsal nucleus. II. Efferent connections. *Brain Res., 12:*321–343, 1969.

Lorente de Nó, R. Studies on the structure of the cerebral cortex. II. Continuation of the study of the Ammonic system. *J. Psychol. Neurol. (Lpz.), 46:*113–177, 1934.

Papez, J.W. A proposed mechanism of emotion. *Arch. Neurol. Psychiat., 38:*725–744, 1937.

Powell, E.W. Limbic projections to the thalamus. *Exp. Brain Res., 17:*394–401, 1973.

Powell, T.P.S. Sensory convergence in the cerebral cortex. In Laitinen, L.V., & Livingston, K.E. (Eds.): *Surgical Approaches in Psychiatry.* Baltimore, University Park Press, 1973.

Rose, J.E., & Woolsey, C.N. Structure and relations of limbic cortex and anterior thalamic nuclei in rabbit and cat. *J. Comp. Neurol., 89:*279–348, 1948.

Chapter 11: Histochemical Mapping of the Limbic System (Pp. 105–115)

The histochemical mapping procedures have provided a whole new approach to descriptive and functional anatomy. These procedures should not be viewed as a replacement of other procedures, but rather as a supplement. Hence, the reader is urged to integrate the references cited below with those of all preceding chapters.

Some useful descriptions of the neurotransmitter systems that form the substrate for these procedures may be found in the following:

Cooper, J.R., Bloom, F.E. & Roth, R.H. *The Biochemical Basis of Neuropharmacology.* New York, Oxford University Press, 1970.

Goodman, L.S., & Gilman, A. *The Pharmacological Basis of Therapeutics.* New York, Macmillan, 1965.

Hall, Z.W., Hildebrand, J.G., & Kravitz, E.A. (Eds.) *Chemistry of Synaptic Transmission.* Newton, Mass., Chiron, 1974.

McLennan, H. *Synaptic Transmission.* Philadelphia, Saunders, 1970.

Rech, R.H., & Moore, K.E. (Eds.) *An Introduction of Psychopharmacology.* New York, Raven, 1971.

Shepherd, G.M. *The Synaptic Organization of the Brain.* New York, Oxford University Press, 1974.

The following articles describe procedures and results of histochemical techniques based on **monoaminergic** transmitter systems:

Aghajanian, G.K., & Gallagher, D.W. Raphe origin of serotonergic nerves terminating in the cerebral ventricles. *Brain Res., 88:*221–231, 1975.

Andén, N.E., Dahlström, A., Fuxe, K., Larsson, K., Olson, L., & Ungerstedt, U. Ascending monoamine neurons to the telencephalon and diencephalon. *Acta Physiol. Scand., 67:*313–326, 1966.

Blackstad, T.W., Fuxe, K., & Hökfelt, T. Noradrenaline nerve terminals in the hippocampal region of the rat and the guinea pig. *Z. Zellforsch. Mikrosk. Anat., 78:*463–473, 1967.

Bloom, F.E. The gains in brain are mainly in the stain. In Worden, F.G., Swazey, J.P., & Adelman, G. *The Neurosciences: Paths of Discovery.* Cambridge, M.I.T. Press, 1975.

Bobbillier, P., Pettijean, F., Salvert, D., Ligier, M., & Seguin, S. Differential projections of the nucleus raphe dorsalis and nucleus ventralis as revealed by autoradiography. *Brain Res., 85:*201–203, 1975.

Carlsson, A., Falck, B., & Hillarp, N.A. Cellular localization of brain monoamines. *Acta Physiol. Scand.,* Suppl. *196:*6–28, 1962.

Clavier, R.M., & Routtenberg, A. Ascending monoamine-containing fiber pathways related to intracranial self-stimulation: histochemical flourescence study. *Brain Res., 72:*25–40, 1974.

Dahlström, A., & Fuxe, K. Evidence for the existence of monoamine-containing neurons in the central nervous system. *Acta Physiol. Scand., 62:*3–55, 1964.

Deguchi, T., Sinha, A.K., & Barchas, J.D. Biosynthesis of serotonin in raphe nuclei of rat brain: effect of p-chlorophenylalanine. *J. Neurochem., 20:*1329–1336, 1973.

Descarries, L., Beaudet, A., & Watkins, K.C. Serotonin nerve terminals in adult rat neocortex. *Brain Res., 100:*563–588, 1975.

Falck, B. Observations on the possibility of the cellular localization of monoamines by a flourescence method. *Acta Physiol. Scand., 56:*6–25, 1962.

Fuxe, K., Goldstein, M., Hökfelt, T., Johnsson, G., & Lidbrink, P. Dopaminergic involvement in hypothalamic function: extra-hypothalamic control. A neuroanatomical analysis. *Adv. Neurol., 5:*405–419, 1974.

Harvey, J.A., Heller, A., Moore, R.Y., Hunt, H.F., & Roth, L.J. Effect of central nervous system lesions on barbiturate sleeping time in the rat. *J. Pharmacol. Exp. Ther., 144:* 24, 1964.

Heller, A., & Moore, R.Y. Effect of central nervous system lesions on brain monoamines in the rat. *J. Pharmacol. Exp. Ther., 150:*1–9, 1965.

Hökfelt, T., Fuxe, K., Goldstein, M., Johansson, O., & Ljungdahl, A. Recent developments in monoamine histochemistry. *J. Psychiat. Res., 11:*277–280, 1974.

Koob, G.F., Balcom, G.J., & Meterhoff, J.L. Dopamine and norepinephrine levels in the nucleus accumbens, olfactory tubercle and corpus striatum following lesions in the ventral tegmental area. *Brain Res., 94:*45–55, 1975.

Kobayashi, R.M., Palkovits, M., Kopin, I.J., & Jacobowitz, D.M. Biochemical mapping of noradrenergic nerves arising from the rat locus coeruleus. *Brain Res., 77:*269–279, 1974.

Kuhar, M.J., Simon, J.R., & Taylor, N. Serotonergic synaptosomes from rat hippocampus: lack of acetylcholinesterase. *Brain Res., 99:*415–418, 1975.

Lindvall, O., & Björklund, A. The organization of the ascending catecholamine neuron systems in the rat brain as revealed by the glyoxylic acid flourescence method. *Acta Physiol. Scand.,* Suppl. *412:*1–48, 1974.

Lorens, S.A., & Guldberg, H.C. Regional 5-hydroxytryptamine following selective midbrain raphe lesions in the rat. *Brain Res., 78:*45–56, 1974.

Lynch, G., Gall, C., Mensah, P., & Cotman, C.W. Horseradish peroxidase histochemistry: a new method for tracing efferent projections in the central nervous system. *Brain Res., 79:*373–380, 1974.

Lynch, G., Smith, R.L., & Robertson, R. Direct projections from brainstem to telencephalon. *Exp. Brain Res., 17:*221–228, 1973.

Moore, R.Y. Brain lesions and monoamine metabolism. *Int. Rev. Neurobiol., 13:*67–91, 1970.

Moore, R.Y., & Halaris, A.E. Hippocampal innervation by serotonin neurons of the midbrain raphe in the rat. *J. Comp. Neurol., 164:*171–183, 1975.

Moore, R.Y., & Heller, A. Monoamine levels and neuronal degeneration in rat brain following lateral hypothalamic lesions. *J. Pharmacol. Exp. Ther., 156:*12–22, 1967.

Moore, R.Y., Wong, S.L.R., & Heller, A. Regional effects of hypothalamic lesions on brain serotonin. *Archiv. Neurol., 13:*346–354, 1965.

Morgane, P.J., & Stern, W.C. Chemical anatomy of brain circuits in relation to sleep and wakefulness. In Weitzman, E.D. (Ed.): *Advances in Sleep Research, Vol. 1.* New York, Spectrum, pp. 1–131, 1974.

Paul, S.M., Heath, R.G., & Ellison, J.P. Histochemical demonstration of a direct pathway from the fastigial nucleus to the septal region. *Exp. Neurol., 40:*798–805, 1973.

Pickel, V.M., Segal, M., & Bloom, F.E. A radioautographic study of the efferent pathways of the nucleus locus coeruleus. *J. Comp. Neurol., 155:*15–42, 1974.

Roizen, M.F., & Jacobowitz, D.M. Studies on the origin of innervation of the noradrenergic area bordering on the nucleus raphe dorsalis. *Brain Res., 101:*561–568, 1976.

Sachs, C., Johnsson, G., & Fuxe, K. Mapping of the central noradrenaline pathways with 6-hydroxy-dopa. *Brain Res., 63:*249–261, 1973.

Simon, H., Lemoal, M., Galey, D., & Cardo, B. Selective degeneration of central dopaminergic systems after injection of 6-hydroxydopamine in the ventral mesencephalic tegmentum of the rat. Demonstration by the Fink-Heimer stain. *Exp. Brain Res., 20:*375–384, 1974.

Swanson, L.W., & Hartman, B.K. The central adrenergic system. An immunoflourescence study of the location of cell bodies and their efferent connections in the rat utilizing dopamine-beta-hydroxylase as a marker. *J. Comp. Neurol., 163:*467–505, 1975.

Toyama, M., Maeda, T., & Shimizu, N. Detailed noradrenaline pathways of locus coeruleus neurons to the cerebral cortex with use of 6-hydroxydopa. *Brain Res., 79:*139–144, 1974.

Ungerstedt, U. Stereotaxic mapping of the monoamine pathways in the rat brain. *Acta Physiol. Scand.,* Suppl. *367:*1–47, 1971.

The following articles describe procedures and results of histochemical mapping procedures that are based on **cholinergic** transmitter systems:

Domino, E.F., Dren, A.T., & Yamamoto, K.I. Pharmacologic evidence for cholinergic mechanisms in neocortical and limbic activating systems. In Adey, W.R., & Tokizane, T. (Eds.): *Progress in Brain Research, Vol. 27.* Amsterdam, Elsevier, pp. 337–363, 1967.

Koelle, G.B. The histochemical localization of cholinesterases in the central nervous system of the rat. *J. Comp. Neurol., 100:*211, 1954.

Lewis, P.R., & Shute, C.C.D. The cholinergic limbic system: projections to hippocampal formation, medial cortex, nuclei of the ascending cholinergic reticular system and the subfornical organ and supraoptic crest. *Brain, 90:*521–539, 1967.

Shute, C.C.D. Cholinergic pathways in the brain. In Laitinen, L.V., & Livingston, K.E. (Eds.): *Surgical Approaches in Psychiatry,* Baltimore, University Park Press, 1973.

Shute, C.C.D., & Lewis, P.R. Cholinesterase-containing systems of the brain of the rat. *Nature, 199:*1160–1164, 1963.

Shute, C.C.D., & Lewis, P.R. The ascending cholinergic reticular system: neocortical, olfactory and subcortical projections. *Brain, 90:*497–521, 1967.

Yamamura, H.I., & Snyder, S.H. Postsynaptic localization of muscarinic cholinergic receptor binding in rat hippocampus. *Brain Res., 78:*320–326, 1974.

Chapter 12: Some Fundamental Approaches to an Analysis of Limbic System Function (Pp. 117–128)

The references listed below include only those cited directly in the text of Chapter 12. Additional references may be found in numerous secondary sources and by cross-referencing with Chapter 3:

Albert, D.J. A simple method of making cuts in brain tissue. *Physiol. Behav.* 4:863–864, 1969.

Anand, B.K., & Brobeck, J.R. Hypothalamic control of food intake in rats and cats. *Yale J. Biol. Med., 24:*123–140, 1951.

Beatty, W.W., & Schwartzbaum, J.S. Enhanced reactivity to quinine and saccharin solutions following septal lesions in the rat. *Psychon. Sci., 8:*483–484, 1968.

Bitterman, M.E. Phyletic differences in learning. *Am. Psychol., 20:*396–410, 1965.

Broca, P. Anatomie comparée des circonvolutions cérébrales. Le grand lobe limbique et la scissure limbique dans la serie des mammifères. *Rev. Anthropol., 1:*385–498, 1878.

Brown, G., & Remley, N. The effects of septal and olfactory bulb lesions on stimulus reactivity. *Physiol. Behav., 6:*497–501, 1971.

Bures, J., Buresova, O., & Fifkova, E. Interhemispheric transfer of a passive avoidance reaction. *J. Comp. Physiol. Psychol., 57*:326–330, 1964.

Campbell, B.A., Lytle, L.D., & Fibiger, H.C. Ontogeny of adrenergic arousal and cholinergic inhibitory mechanisms in the rat. *Science, 166*:635–637, 1969.

Carlton, P.L. Cholinergic mechanisms in the control of behavior by the brain. *Psychol. Rev. 40*:19–39, 1963.

Carlton, P.L. Brain acetylcholine and inhibition. In Tapp, J. (Ed.): *Reinforcement and Behavior*, New York, Academic Press, pp. 288–325, 1969.

Carlton, P.L., & Advokat, C. Attenuated habituation due to parachlorophenylalanine. *Pharmacol. Biochem. Behav., 1*:657–663, 1974.

Clark, G. The use of the Horsely-Clark instrument on the rat. *Science, 90*:92, 1939.

Cooper, J.R., Bloom, F.E., & Roth, R.H. *The Biochemical Basis of Neuropharmacology*. New York, Oxford University Press, 1970.

Crow, T.J. Catecholamine containing neurons and electrical self-stimulation. 1. A review of some data. *Psychol. Med., 2*:414–421, 1972.

Feigley, D.A. Effects of scopolamine on activity and passive avoidance learning in rats of different ages. *J. Comp. Physiol. Psychol., 87*:26–36, 1974.

Feigley, D.A., Parsons, P.J., Hamilton, L.W., & Spear, N.E. Development of habituation to novel environments in the rat. *J. Comp. Physiol. Psychol., 79*:443–452, 1972.

Fritsch, G., & Hitzig, E. Über die elektrische Erregbarkeit des Grosshirns. *Arch. Anat. Physiol. Wissen. Med., 37*:300–332, 1870.

Goodman, L.S., & Gilman, A. *The Pharmacological Basis of Therapeutics*. New York. Macmillan, 1965.

Gottlieb, G. Ontogenesis of sensory function in birds and mammals. In Tobach, E., Aronson, L.R., & Shaw, E. (Eds.): *Biopsychology of Development*, New York. Academic Press, pp. 67–128, 1971.

Grossman, S.P. Behavioral effects of direct chemical stimulation of central nervous system structures. *Int. J. Neuropharmacol., 3*:45–58, 1964.

Grossman, S.P. *A Textbook of Physiological Psychology*. New York, Wiley, 1967.

Halasz, B., & Pupp, L. Hormone secretion of the anterior pituitary gland after physical interruption of all nervous pathways to the hypophysiotropic area. *Endocrinology, 77*:553–562, 1965.

Hamilton, L.W., & Timmons, C.R. Knife cuts while you wait: a simple and inexpensive procedure for producing knife cuts in freely moving animals. *Physiol. Behav., 16*:101–103, 1976.

Hamilton, L.W., Capobianco, S., & Worsham, E. Lowered response to postingestive cues following septal lesions in rats. *J. Comp. Physiol. Psychol., 87*:134–141, 1974.

Hamilton, L.W., Worsham, E., & Capobianco, S. A spring-loaded carrier for transection of fornix and other large fiber bundles. *Physiol. Behav., 10*:157–159, 1973.

Harlow, H.F., Blomquist, A.J., Thompson, C.I., Schiltz, K.A., & Harlow, M.K. Effects of induction age and size of frontal lobe lesions on learning in rhesus monkeys. In Isaacson, R.L. (Ed.): *The Neuropsychology of Development*, New York, Wiley, pp. 79–120, 1968.

Hetherington, A.W., & Ranson, S.W. Hypothalamic lesions and adiposity in the rat. *Anat. Rec., 78*:149, 1940.

Horsely, V., & Clark, R.H. The structure and functions of the cerebellum examined by a new method. *Brain, 31*:45–124, 1908.

Isaacson, R.L. *The Limbic System*, New York, Plenum Press, 1974.

Isaacson, R.L., Nonneman, A.J., & Schmaltz, L.W. Behavioral and anatomical sequelae of the infant limbic system. In Isaacson, R.L. (Ed.): *The Neuropsychology of Development*, New York, Wiley, pp. 41–78, 1968.

Jouvet, M. The role of monoamines and acetylcholine-containing neurons in the regulation of the sleep-waking cycle. *Ergeb. Physiol., 64*:166–307, 1972.

Kaada, B.R. Somato-motor, autonomic and electroencephalographic responses to electrical stimulation of "rhinencephalic" and other forebrain structures in primates, cat and dog. *Acta Physiol. Scand., 83*:1–285, 1951.

Krauthamer, G.M. Catecholamines in behavior and sensorimotor integration: the neostriatal system. In Friedhoff, A.J., *Catecholamines and Behavior*, New York, Plenum Press, pp. 59–87, 1975.

MacLean, P.D. Some psychiatric implications of physiological studies of fronto-temporal portion of limbic system (visceral brain). *Electoeneephalog. Clin. Neurophysiol., 4*:407–418, 1952.

MacLean, P.D. The triune brain, emotion and scientific bias. In Schmidt, F.O. (Ed.): *The Neurosciences Second Study Program*, New York, Rockefeller University Press, pp. 336–348, 1970.

Mabry, P.D., & Campbell, B.A. Ontogeny of serotonergic inhibition of behavioral arousal in the rat. *J. Comp. Physiol. Psychol., 86*:193–201, 1974.

Mandel, P., Mack, G., & Goridis, C. Function of the central catecholaminergic neuron: synthesis, release, and inactivation of the transmitter. In Friedhoff, A.J. (Ed.): *Catecholamines and Behavior,* New York, Plenum Press, 1975.

McCleary, R.A. Response specificity in the behavioral effects of limbic system lesions in the cat. *J. Comp. Physiol. Psychol., 54:*605–613, 1961.

McCleary, R.A. Response-modulating functions of the limbic system: initiation and suppression. In Stellar, E., & Sprague, J.M. (Eds.): Progress in Physiological Psychology, Vol. 1. New York, Academic Press, 1966.

McLennan, H. *Synaptic Transmission.* Philadelphia, Saunders, 1970.

Milner, P.M. *Physiological Psychology.* New York, Holt, Rinehart & Winston, 1970.

Myers, R.D. *Methods in Psychobiology.* London, Academic, 1972.

Nauta, W.J.H. Hippocampal projections and related neural pathways to the midbrain in the cat. *Brain, 81:*319–340, 1958.

Nauta, W.J.H. Connections of the frontal lobe with the limbic system. In Laitinen, L.V., & Livingston, K.E. (Eds.): *Surgical Approaches in Psychiatry,* Baltimore, University Park Press, 1973.

Papez, J.W. A proposed mechanism of emotion. *Arch. Neurol. Psychiat., 38:*725–743, 1937.

Penfield, W., & Rasmussen, T. *The Cerebral Cortex of Man.* New York, Macmillan, 1950.

Pribram, K.H., & Kruger, L. Functions of the "olfactory brain." *Ann. N.Y. Acad Sci., 58:*109–138, 1954.

Robinson, B.W. Forebrain alimentary responses: some organizational principles. In Wayner, M.J. (Ed.): *Thrist: First International Symposium on Thirst in the Regulation of Body Water,* New York, Pergamon, 1964.

Schoenfeld, T.A., & Hamilton, L.W. Secondary brain changes following lesions: a new paradigm for lesion experimentation. *Physiol. Behav.,* 9177, in press.

Schoenfeld, T.A., Hamilton, L.W., & Gandelman, R. Septal damage during the maturation of inhibitory responding: effects in juvenile and adult rats. *Devel. Psychobiol., 7:*195–205, 1974.

Sclafani, A., & Grossman, S.P. Hyperphagia produced by knife cuts between the medial and lateral hypothalamus in the rat. *Physiol. Behav., 4:*533–537, 1969.

Shute, C.C.D., & Lewis, P.R. The ascending cholinergic reticular system: neocortical, olfactory and subcortical projections. *Brain, 90:*497–522, 1967.

Stein, L. Chemistry of reward and punishment. In Efron, D.H. (Ed.): *Psychopharmacology: A Review of Progress, 1957–1967,* U.S.P.H.S., pp. 105–123, 1968.

Wiess, B., & Laties, V.G. Enhancement of human performance by caffeine and the amphetamines. *Pharmacol. Rev., 14:*1–1962.

Williams, J.M., Hamilton, L.W., & Carlton, P.L. An ontogenetic analysis of two classes of habituation. *J. Comp. Physiol. Psychol., 89:*733–737, 1975.

White, B.C. Effects of hippocampal lesions on reversal and passive avoidance learning: an ontogenetic study. A paper presented to the Eastern Psychological Association, Boston, Massachusetts, 1972.

White, B.C., & McGee, S.A. Personal communication.

PART II: REFERENCE SOURCES

Rat Brain Atlases

Albe-Gessard, D., Stutinsky, F. & Libouban, S. *Atlat stéréotaxique du Diencéphale du Rat Blanc.* Editions CNRS, Paris, 1966.

Bernardis, L.L., & Skelton, F.R. Stereotaxic localization of supraoptic, ventromedial and mammillary nuclei in the hypothalamus of weanling and mature rats. *Am. J. Anat., 116:*69–74, 1965.

de Groot, J. *The Rat Forebrain in Stereotaxic Coordinates.* Amsterdam, The Netherlands, Verhandlingen der koninklijke Nederlanse Akademie van Wetenschappen, Afd. Naturekunde, N. V. Noord-Hollandsche Uitgevers Maatschappij, 1959.

Fifkova, E., & Marsala, J. Stereotaxic atlases for the cat, rabbit, and rat. In Bureš, J., Petráň, M., & Zachar, J. (Eds.): *Electrophysiological Methods in Biological Research,* New York, Academic Press, pp. 653–731, 1967.

König, J.F.R., & Klippel, R.A. *The Rat Brain: A Stereotaxic Atlas of the Forebrain and Lower Parts of the Brainstem.* Baltimore, Williams & Wilkins, 1963.

Krieg, W.J.S. Accurate placement of minute lesions in the brain of the albino rat. *Quart. Bull. Northwestern Univ. Med. School, 20:*199–208, 1946.

Massopust, L.C. Diencephalon of the rat. In Sheer, D.E. (Ed.): *Electrical Stimulation of the Brain,* Austin, University of Texas Press, pp. 182–202, 1961.

Pellegrino, L.J., & Cushman, A.J. *A Stereotaxic Atlas of the Rat Brain*. New York, Appleton-Century-Crofts, 1967.

Sherwood, M.S., & Timirias, P.S. *A Stereotaxic Atlas of the Developing Rat Brain*. Berkeley, University of California Press, 1970.

Zeman, W., & Innes, J.R.M. *Craigie's Neuroanatomy of the Rat*. New York, Academic Press, 1963.

An exhaustive list of atlases may be obtained from David Kopf Instruments, 7324 Elmo Street, Tujunga, Cal. 91042.

Textbooks of Neuroanatomy

Some of the major textbooks of neuroanatomy (mostly dealing with human brains) are listed below:

Bossy, J. *Atlas of Neuroanatomy and Special Sense Organs*. Philadelphia, Saunders, 1970.

Carpenter, M.B. *Core Text of Neuroanatomy*. Baltimore, Williams & Wilkins, 1972.

Chusid, J.G. *Correlative Neuroanatomy and Functional Neurology*. Los Altos, Cal., Lange Medical Publications, 1973.

Crosby, E.C., Humphrey, T., & Lauer, E.W. *Correlative Anatomy of the Nervous System*. New York, Macmillan, 1962.

von Economo, C. *The Cytoarchitectonics of the Human Cerebral Cortex* (trans.). New York, Oxford University Press, 1929.

Gardner, E. *Fundamentals of Neurology*. Philadelphia, Saunders, 1963.

Kappers, C.U.A., Huber, G.C., & Crosby, E.C. *The Comparative Anatomy of the Nervous System of Vertebrates*. New York, Macmillan, 1936.

Holmes, R.L. *The Human Nervous System: A Developmental Approach*. London, Churchill, 1969.

House, L., & Pansky, B. *A Functional Approach to Neuroanatomy*. New York, McGraw-Hill, 1967.

Jenkins, T.W. *Functional Mammalian Neuroanatomy, with Emphasis on Dog and Cat, Including an Atlas of Dog Central Nervous System*. Philadelphia, Lea & Febiger, 1972.

Netter, F.H. *The Ciba Collection of Medical Illustrations. Vol. I. Nervous System*. Summit, N.J., Ciba Pharmaceutical Products Co., 1953.

Noback, C.R., & Demarest, R.J. *The Human Nervous System*. New York, McGraw-Hill, 1975.

Ranson, S.W., & Clark, S.L. *The Anatomy of the Nervous System*. Philadelphia, Saunders, 1959.

Sidman, R.L., & Sidman, M. *Neuroanatomy: A Programmed Text*. Boston, Little, Brown & Co., 1965.

Truex, R.C. *Human Neuroanatomy*. Baltimore, Williams & Wilkins, 1969.

Technical Journals

Major technical journals that are likely to publish recent research on limbic system anatomy, function, and development include:

Anatomical Record
Behavioral Biology
Brain
Brain Research
Developmental Psychobiology
Electroencephalography and Clinical Neurophysiology
Experimental Neurology
International Reviews of Neurobiology
Journal of Comparative Neurology
Journal of Comparative and Physiological Psychology
Journal of Pharmacology and Experimental Therapeutics
Physiological Reviews
Physiological Psychology
Physiology, Biochemistry and Behavior
Physiology and Behavior
Psychological Reviews

Author Index

145

Structure Index

147

STRUCTURE INDEX